# 365 Days

## Of

## KETOGENIC

## &

## ANTI-AGING

## DIETS

*495 Easy to prepare Keto & Anti-Aging Meals*

*(Vol.2)*

## SANDRA WOODS

# Contents

**Contents**

i

# Copyright

ISBN-13: 978-1981841073

ISBN-10: 1981841075

# Dedication

*This book is dedicated to all lovers of healthy meals and those who are not satisfied until they learn new ways of preparing one.*

*"You learn to cook so that you don't have to be a slave to recipes. You get what's in season and you know what to do with it"*

- Julia Child

# CHAPTER ONE

## *Introduction*

There are several books out there on ketogenic dieting, however, this is different from most of the books you have ever read on this topic because it doesn't just talk about ketogenic diets, but diets that contains antioxidant to slow down aging drastically.

Our skin is a reflection of what we consume as food and this goes a long way to decide if our skin would remain smooth for a long time to come or starts sagging. This book is meant for both keto beginners as well as advance keto users. Each of the diet in this book is outlines all the dietary content to serve as a guide for you to know the amount of calories you would consume when you prepare each meal.

That burning sensation in your chest after climbing up two flights of stairs, your skin wrinkling so fast, jeans that don't fit, and friends that tell you "I think you're getting chubby,"— are you getting a bit tired of these? Are you in dire need of losing those excess pounds you've carried around since Thanksgiving three years ago?

Right now, maybe you're feeling awful about your weight and physical appearance, but let me tell you this: the moment that you decided that you need to do something about your dilemma (like purchasing this book), means you're already halfway to losing weight, improving your health, and becoming a better version of you.

But before I introduce this effective and revolutionary diet that will help solve your problems, let's straighten a few things up. Let me ask you a few fundamental questions that may just shift your perspective:

What is the real reason why you want to shed the fat and lose weight? Is it to boost your confidence and have the perfect bikini body? Or is it so that you can run that marathon you have always wanted to?

You see, there's nothing wrong with wanting to lose weight in order to become more attractive, but should this be your main focus? This may be your initial goal, but after committing to the Ketogenic lifestyle you will soon realize that the benefits are far more extensive than just mere weight loss.

Mood stabilization, hormone regulation, slowed ageing, blood sugar balance, memory and cognitive improvement these are just a few of the profound changes your body will embrace should you choose to follow the advice that is contained in the pages to follow.

So, besides achieving a "desirable" body, your main purpose will rapidly shift to becoming a healthy, energetic person, avoiding the severe complications of being overweight or obese. Experts have recognized that the primary cause of these conditions is a deadly combination of an unhealthy diet, plus a sedentary lifestyle.

It is quite disturbing to note that over 1.9 billion adults all over the world are suffering these conditions (WHO, 2014); 42 million children below 5 years old are also either obese or overweight.

Now you might be asking: How does this affect me? Well, carrying extra pounds around your mid-section puts you at great risk of developing chronic illnesses such as stroke, heart disease, type 2 diabetes, osteoarthritis, breast cancer and colon cancer, just to name a few. Although these complications may alarm you, the good news is that obesity can be reversed and the complications that go with it are preventable.

The simplest answer is invariably the correct one, and you have most likely heard it a thousand times before. A balanced diet mixed with a healthy dose of exercise. The first part of the statement is where most individuals slip up. The so called "balance diet" is never fully explained and always shrouded in mystery and confusion.

Maybe you've already tried some of the fad diets that are popular right now, but they do not seem to work. Or you have also tried some of the fasting and starvation diets out there that promise instant results, but you just can't seem to keep up with the idea of skipping meals. Well, maybe it's time that you try a diet that is scientifically proven to help you burn fat, lose weight, and provide you much, much more - the Ketogenic Diet.

Also, called the Keto Diet, this food program is a low-carb high-fat diet that "forces" the body to enter into a different metabolic state where fat is burned as fuel for energy instead of glucose (I will discuss this in more detail at a later stage in the book). You may think that the Keto Diet is a fairly new food regimen, yet another fad, but on the contrary, this diet has already become popular in the 1940's when it was used to help minimize epileptic related seizures of children.

It has since lost its place under the spotlight when anticonvulsant drugs became more widely available to the market. It only gained popularity again in the 1990's, when the son of a famous Hollywood director used the diet to help him reduce his epileptic episodes, with remarkable results.

This paved way for further research into the Keto-based Diets. These studies found that a low-carb, high-fat diet was not only able to help minimize seizures for patients with epilepsy, but also help individuals to lose weight, minimize abdominal fat, increase HDL and LDL levels (good cholesterol), decrease blood sugar levels, prevent cancer and cognitive decline. So, in short, this diet that I'm about to introduce to you will not only help you burn fat and lose weight, but it can also deliver other amazing benefits for your overall health!

Before I go any further, I'd like to thank and congratulate you for purchasing this book. This book will help you and understand what the Ketogenic Diet is and how you can use it to lose weight—fast! The chapters of this book will provide you with the information on how you can start transitioning into ketosis and how to create your own Keto meal plan. I will also provide a comprehensive list of Ketogenic approved foods. I've also included delicious Keto recipes for breakfast, lunch, dinner and snacks. Most importantly, I've included a 4-week Keto eating plan that can help guide you on your first month in the Keto Diet. Today is a beginning of a better and healthier you!

This book is a two-series book, for you to get the complete 365 days recipes, you would please need to purchase the First volume.

## How to Get Started: Transitioning into Ketosis

You've heard of countless low-carb diets that help you lose weight and at the same time deliver amazing health benefits, but a low-carb high-fat diet? How does that work? How can eating more fat, help you lose fat? Well, that is where the metabolic processes ketosis steps in to help out.

## The "Standard American Diet" vs. Keto Diet

Ever since modern agriculture was introduced, man's normal diet has shifted from being meat and vegetable eaters (our hunter and gatherer ancestors) to individuals who eat more processed carbohydrates such as pasta, bread, rice, and potatoes.

Now, there's nothing wrong with carbs. Carbs per se isn't actually bad for our health as long as we consume more of the healthy types of carbs such as vegetables (yes they contain carbs too), legumes, whole-grains, fruits, and nuts.

However, if you really want to lose weight and also prevent developing type 2 diabetes, then it would be advisable to limit a number of carbs you consume. That's because when you eat foods high in carbohydrates they get broken down in your blood as glucose (sugar). This means that when you consume lots of carbs, a high amount of glucose becomes present in your blood, resulting in high blood sugar levels.

Again, carbs aren't all bad because in a normal diet the body will reach out for glucose in order to use it as fuel for energy, as well as fuel the other functions of our body. The only problem is that any glucose that isn't used by the body as energy will be stored as body fat. This is one of the main reasons why a lot of people in today's day and age are overweight - because they consume too many carbs and only expend little of it due to their sedentary lifestyle.

The Ketogenic Diet, on the other hand, reduces the consumption of carbs to a minimum and increases healthy fats in one's diet. When carbs are reduced, your body will naturally look for other sources to burn for energy and in this case, fats are chosen. The Ketogenic Diet shifts your body into a metabolic state called ketosis, a process that burns fat instead of glucose allowing you to shed unwanted weight easily and quickly.

## *Entering Ketosis*

As you now know, the target of the Ketogenic Diet is to allow your body to enter into ketosis; but the question now is, how?

There are three different types of Ketogenic Diets— the Standard Ketogenic Diet (SKD), Cyclical Ketogenic Diet (CKD), and the Targeted Ketogenic Diet (TKD). The latter two variants of the diet will be ignored due to their complexity. People who have sedentary lifestyles and wish to lose weight through this diet are advised to follow the SKD.

This variation recommends limiting the consumption of your carbs to 20-50 grams daily, which means your macronutrients should be made up of 70%-75% fat, 20%-25% protein, and 5%-10% carbs. The number of daily calories you can consume, however, relies on your weight, height, age, and activity. If you're unsure how to do this, you can always consult a keto calculator, which are widely available online.

You might be a little skeptical of the Ketogenic Diet right now, especially if you think that carbs currently make up the biggest portion of your diet. Set aside your assumptions for the duration of this book and approach the next two weeks of your life like an experiment. Trust that if you consume a healthy number of calories and eat foods that are nutrient dense (ex. vegetables, and healthy fat), then you don't have to worry about "dieting" at all! You can safely enter into a state of ketosis when following the prescribed guidelines closely.

I'd like to remind you that unlike any other diets, the Keto Diet needs your complete commitment to the diet in order for you to achieve the state of ketosis. Depending on your body type, activity level, and your diet, you can get into ketosis anywhere from 2 days to a week. For beginners, it is advisable that you use urine ketone sticks (such as Ketostix) to monitor the levels of ketones in your body and ensure that you are in ketosis state. This is a useful tip to help you know whether your body is in ketosis and is burning fat as energy, apart from the other obvious indicators like an increase in energy and lack of appetite.

I must advise you, however, that before anything else, it is a must that you ask for a green light from your health care provider if you are planning to follow the Ketogenic Diet; or any type of diet for that matter. Although this diet is over-all safe, even for kids, you have to let your doctor know about this especially if you have existing health conditions.

Pregnant women or those who are breastfeeding aren't encouraged to try the Ketogenic Diet for weight loss because this may have adverse effects on their baby.

# Approved Ketosis Recipes

Time to purge your pantry and replace them with these Ketogenic Diet approved foods!

*Fats and Oils*

Since fat will make the majority of your meals, it is a must that you choose the good type  (natural sources) of fat and not those that are dangerous to your health. Some of your best choices for fat are:

Ghee or Clarified butter

Avocado

Coconut Oil

Red Palm Oil

Butter

Coconut Butter

Peanut Butter

Chicken Fat

Beef Tallow

Non-hydrogenated Lard

Macadamia Nuts

Egg Yolks


Fish rich in Omega-3 Fatty Acids like salmon,  mackerel, trout,  tuna, and even shellfish.

*Protein*

In order to achieve a state of ketosis, you need to consume 20%-25% protein in your daily caloric allowance. This means your consumption of fat will be high; carbs are low, and protein, moderate. Of course, you also want to choose the healthy sources of protein that are either organic, or grass fed.

Meat— beef, veal, lamb, chicken, duck, pheasant, pork chops, pork loin, etc.

Deli Meat— bacon, sausage, ham (make sure to watch out of added sugar and other fillers)

Eggs— preferably free-range or organic eggs

Fish— wild caught salmon, catfish, halibut, trout, tuna, etc.

Seafood— lobster, crab, oyster, clams, mussels

Peanut Butter—this is a great source of protein, but make sure to choose the all-natural variant.

*Dairy*

Compared to other weight loss diets, in the Ketogenic Diet, you are encouraged to choose dairy products that are full fat. Some of the best dairy products that you can choose are:

Hard and Soft Cheese— cream cheese, mozzarella, cheddar, etc.

Cottage Cheese

Heavy Whipping Cream

Sour Cream

Full-Fat Yogurt

*Vegetables*

Overall, vegetables are rich in vitamins and minerals that contribute to a healthy body. However, if you're aiming to avoid carbs, it's best that you keep away from starchy vegetables such as potatoes, yam, peas, corn, beans, and legumes. You also want to limit vegetables that taste sweet such as carrots and squash. Instead, stick with green leafy vegetables that are preferably organically grown and other low-carb veggies.

Spinach

Lettuce

Collard Greens

Mustard Greens

Bok Choi

Kale

Alfalfa Sprouts

Celery

Tomato

Broccoli

Cauliflower

eat occasionally

*Fruits*

Your choice of fruit is only limited to avocado and some *berries because fruits are high in carbs and sugar.

*Drinks*

Water

Black Coffee

Herbal Tea

Wine—white wine and dry red wine are OK, as long as they are only consumed occasionally.

*Others*

Homemade Mayo—if you want to buy mayo from the store, make sure that you watch out for the hidden carbs it contains

Homemade Mustard

Any type of Spices and Herbs

Honey

Stevia

Agave Nectar

Ketchup (Sugar-free)

Dark Chocolate/Cocoa

Food List by Color

*Green List*

This is an all-you-can-eat list - you choose anything you like without worrying about the carbohydrate content as all the foods will be between 0 to 5g/100g.

It will be almost impossible to overdo your carbohydrate intake by sticking to this group of foods. Eating large amounts of protein is not recommended, so eat a moderate amount of animal protein at each meal. Include as much fat as you are comfortable with - bearing in mind that Keto is high in fat. Caution: even though these are all-you-can-eat foods, only eat when hungry, stop when full and do not overeat. The size and thickness of your palm without fingers is a good measure for a serving of animal protein. All meat, eggs, dairy, and greens should be organic, free range and grass fed where possible.

*Animal Protein*

(unless these have a rating, they are all 0g/100g)

All eggs

All meats, poultry, and game

All natural and cured meats (pancetta, parma ham, capocollo etc)

All natural and cured sausages (salami, chorizo etc)

All offal

All seafood (except swordfish and tilefish - high mercury content)

Broths

*Dairy*

Cottage cheese

Cream

Cream cheese

Full-cream Greek yogurt

Full-cream milk

Hard cheeses

Soft cheeses

*Fats*

Any rendered animal fat

Avocado oil

Butter

Cheese - firm, natural, full-fat, aged cheeses (not processed)

Coconut oil

Duck fat

Ghee

Lard

Macadamia oil

Mayonnaise, full fat only  (not from seeds oils)

Olive oil

*Flavorings and Condiments*

All flavorings and condiments are okay, provided they do not contain sugars and preservatives or vegetable (seed) oils.

*Nuts and Seeds*

Almonds

Flaxseeds (watch out for pre-ground flax seeds, they go rancid quickly and become toxic)

Macadamia nuts

Pecan nuts

Pine nuts

Pumpkin seeds

Sunflower seeds

Walnuts

SWEETENERS

Erythritol granules

Stevia powder

Xylitol granules

*Vegetables*

All green leafy vegetables (spinach, cabbage, lettuces etc)

Any other vegetables which are grown above the ground (except butternut)

Artichoke hearts

Asparagus

Aubergines

Avocados

Broccoli

Brussels sprouts

Cabbage

Cauliflower

Celery

Courgettes

Leeks

Mushrooms

Olives

Onions

Peppers

Pumpkin

Radishe

Sauerkraut

Spring onions

Tomatoes

Orange List

Chart your carbohydrates without getting obsessive and still obtain an excellent outcome. If you are endeavoring to go into ketosis, this list will assist you to stay under a total of 50g carbs for the day. These are all net carbs and they are all 23 to 25g per indicated amount. Ingredients are all fresh unless otherwise indicated.

*Fruits*

Apples 1.5

Bananas 1 small

Blackberries 3.5 C

Blueberries 1.5 C

Cherries (sweet) 1 C

Clementine's 3

Figs 3 small

Gooseberries 1.5 C

Grapes (green) less than 1 C

Guavas 2

Kiwi fruits 3

Litchis 18

Mangos, sliced, under 1 C

Nectarines 2

Oranges 2

Pawpaw 1

Peaches 2

Pears (Bartlett) 1

Pineapple, sliced, 1 C

Plums 4

Pomegranate ½

Prickly pears 4

Quinces 2

Raspberries 2

Strawberries 25

Watermelon 2 C

*Nuts*

Cashews, raw, 6 T

Chestnuts, raw, 1 C

*Sweeteners*

Honey 1 t

VEGETABLES

Butternut 1.5 C

Carrots 5

Sweet potato 0.5 C

KEY

C = cups per day

T = tablespoons per day

t = teaspoons per day

g = grams per day

For example, 1.5 apples are all the carbs you can have off the orange list for the day (if you want to go into ketosis and make sure you are under 50g total carbs for the day).

Red will contain all the foods to avoid as they will be either toxic (e.g. seed oils, soya) or high-carbohydrate foods (e.g. potatoes, rice).

We strongly suggest you avoid all the items on this list, or, at best, eat them very occasionally and restrict the amount when you do. They will do nothing to help you in your attempt to reach your goal.

*Baked Goods*

All flours from grains - wheat flour, corn flour, rye flour, barley flour, pea flour, rice flour etc

All forms of bread

All grains - wheat, oats, barley, rye, amaranth, quinoa, teff etc

Beans (dried)

"Breaded" or battered foods

Brans

Breakfast cereals, muesli, granola of any kind

Buckwheat

Cakes, biscuits, confectionery

Corn products - popcorn, polenta, corn thins, maize

Couscous

Crackers, cracker bread

Millet

Pasta, noodles

Rice

Rice cakes

Sorghum

Spelt

Thickening agents such as gravy powder, maize starch or stock cubes

*Beverages*

Beer, cider

Fizzy drinks (sodas) of any description other than carbonated water

Lite, zero, diet drinks of any description

*Dairy / Dairy-Related*

Cheese spreads, commercial spreads

Coffee creamers

Commercial almond milk

Condensed milk

Fat-free anything

Ice cream

Puddings

Reduced-fat cow's milk

Rice milk

Soy milk

*Fats*

All seed oils (safflower, sunflower, canola, grapeseed, cottonseed, corn)

Chocolate

Commercial sauces, marinades, and salad dressings

Hydrogenated or partially hydrogenated oils including margarine, vegetable oils, vegetable fats.


## Creating Your Own Meal Plan

Remember that in order to lose weight on the Ketogenic Diet, you have to let your body enter into the metabolic state of ketosis. Without this, your body will still continue to burn glucose as fuel and would store as fat any excess sugar that isn't used as fuel. In order for you to enter ketosis, you have to decrease your consumption of carbs, increase your intake of fat, and moderately eat protein.

As you know, the foods you eat are key to reset your body and shift you into a different metabolic state. This is why it is very important that you create your own meal plan so that you are sure that everything you eat will not disrupt your metabolism's state of ketosis. My advice is that you determine the macros that you need to consume through the use of this keto calculator so that you can achieve weight loss through the diet.

After you have identified the number of grams of macronutrients (carbs, protein & fat) that you should consume daily for your body type, stick with this number when you create your meal plan.

For example, John, who is an average 6-foot tall male who weighs 190 lbs. (86.2 kg) and lives a sedentary lifestyle. According to the keto calculator, in order for John to lose weight and enter ketosis, he must maintain a daily diet of 1654 kcal made with 25g carbs (6%), 91g protein (22%), and 132g fat (72%).

With these numbers— 1654 calories, 25g net carbs, 91g protein, and 132g fat, John should create a meal plan to help him achieve this.

I've provided you with a meal plan in the next chapter of this book that you can use in the early weeks of your Ketogenic Diet, or you can also create a meal plan of your own using the following tips: Helpful Tips for the Ketogenic Diet

*Learn to Count Your Net Carbs*— As you now know, the key to entering a state of ketosis is to limit your carbs to 20-50 grams (net carbs) every day. One of the useful tools to help you monitor this is through the use of an app called MyFitnessPal (I encourage you to download this on your device!). With this app, you can easily log your foods which can help you monitor the foods you consume.

Although this app doesn't provide you with your consumption of net carbs, it will provide you with the fiber and carbs that you have consumed. To get your net carbs, just simply subtract the fiber from the carbs you consumed.

Beware of Hidden Carbs— It will be very easy for you to avoid foods such as pasta and bread because you know that they contain loads of carbs. However, what most people fail to do is to also count the carbs that are "hidden" in foods such as baked beans, salad dressing, and tomato sauce which all have carbs in them! So, make sure to read labels and count all carbs to stick to the 20-50 grams daily and achieve ketosis.

*Choose the Right Foods*— Even if the Ketogenic Diet is a low-carb high-fat diet, this doesn't give you the liberty to consume as much fat as you can. Choosing the right fats (the saturated kind) is key. Stay from carbs such as pasta, bread, rice and sugar completely. It's just not worth risking it. The 20-50 grams of carbs that you're allowed to consume should be made of nutrient dense vegetables that also have carbs in them.

*Limit Your Consumption of Fruit—* We all know that fruits have loads of vitamins, fiber, and other nutrients that are good for the body. However, if you want to reset your metabolism and allow it to use fat as fuel instead of glucose, then you must limit your consumption of fruit to a minimum. That's because all fruits are high in fructose (a type of sugar), which causes your insulin levels to spike. When that happens, the fats cells in your body are locked and your body will use glucose as energy.

Remember that on the Ketogenic Diet, you are only allowed to have 25-50 grams of net carbs a day. A medium-sized banana already amounts to 24g net carbs, which means, you almost have already consumed all your carbs for the day in just eating a banana. If you still want to consume fruits, you can stick with a cup of mixed berries that has 5g net carbs, but this is not recommended to be consumed daily.

Spend More Time in the Kitchen— For you to achieve ketosis, it is vital that you watch over the foods you eat. That's why it is advisable if you prepare your own meals and avoid eating out too much. Yes, you will have to sacrifice a bit of your time in preparing your meals, but this assures you that you're only consuming what is approved in the Ketogenic Diet.

*About the Recipes*

I have provided an extensive recipe library in the next section as well as an example meal plan to help you whip up your own Keto-approved meals in your kitchen.

The recipes are categorized as follows:

4 Week Keto Meal Plan

| *Meal Plan – Week One* | | | |
|---|---|---|---|
| | *Monday* | *Tuesday* | *Wednesday* |
| *Breakfast* | *Red Pepper, Mozzarella and Bacon Frittata* | *Breakfast Quiche* | *Mahón Kale Sausage Omelet Pie* |
| *Lunch* | *Asian Grilled Chicken* | *Creamy Haddock* | *Cheesy Crust Pizza* |
| *Dinner* | *Chorizo Stuffed Bell Peppers* | *Italian Gnocchi Soup* | *Bouillabaisse Fish Stew* |

| Thursday | Friday | Saturday | Sunday |
|---|---|---|---|
| Hot n' Spicy Scramble | Breakfast Bread Pudding | Chia Flour Pancakes | Keto Baked Pancetta and Eggs |
| Rosemary, Chicken Sausage Pies | Chorizo Stuffed Bell Peppers | Lime Avocado Salmon | Meaty Bagels |
| Stir Fried Beef | Spicy Bacon-Wrapped Dogs | Monterey Jack Steak | Balsamic Pork |

### Meal Plan – Week Two

| | Monday | Tuesday | Wednesday |
|---|---|---|---|
| **Breakfast** | Keto French Almond Toast | Quick Coconut Berry Pancakes | Keto Pork and Sage Breakfast Burgers |
| **Lunch** | Savoury Mince | Baked Creamy | Leftover Meat Salad |

|  |  | Cauliflower-Broccoli Chicken |  |
|---|---|---|---|
| Dinner | Mediterranean Chicken | Pulled Pork Shoulder | Keto Friendly Sushi |
| Thursday | Friday | Saturday | Sunday |
| Millet Gingerbread Mash | Egg Whites and Spinach Omelet | Hemp Muffins with Walnuts | Baked Ham and Kale Scrambled Eggs |
| Shrimp & Avocado Salad | Spring Roll in a Bowl | Cheese Steak Salad | Turkey Meatballs |
| Chicken Parmesan | Baked Pork Chops in Sweet-Sour Marinade | Salmon Burgers | Chicken Satay |

## Meal Plan – Week Three

|  | Monday | Tuesday | Wednesday |
|---|---|---|---|
| Breakfast | Fast Protein and Peanut-Butter Pancakes | Vesuvius Scrambled Eggs with Provolone | Keto Oatmeal |
| Lunch | Chicken Pot Pie | Mackerel Salad | Spicy Mexican Meatballs |
| Dinner | Baked Glazed Salmon | Zesty Herbed Chicken | Sweet and Sour Snapper |

| Thursday | Friday | Saturday | Sunday |
|---|---|---|---|
| Crimini Mushroom with Boiled Eggs Breakfast | Anchovy, Spinach and Asparagus Omelet | Guacamole Bacon and Eggs Breakfast | Keto Bilberry Coconut Mush |

| Salmon Salad in Avo Cups | Creamy Chicken Salad | Bell Peppers Stuffed | Cheeseburger Casserole |
|---|---|---|---|
| Pordenone Cauliflower Lasagna | Lemon Mustard Pork Loin | Seared RibeyeSteak | Macadamia Crusted Lamb Chops |

| Meal Plan – Week Four | | | |
|---|---|---|---|
| | Monday | Tuesday | Wednesday |
| Breakfast | Chocó Mocha Chia Porridge | Keto Pancakes and Syrup | Mediterranean Egg Scramble |
| Lunch | Chicken and Broccoli filled Zucchini | Cheesy Bacon Spinach Log | Meatballs in Coconut Broth |

| Dinner | Lamb Curry & Spinach | Slow-Cooker Stroganoff | Bolognese Squash Spaghetti |
|---|---|---|---|
| Thursday | Friday | Saturday | Sunday |
| Chorizo Breakfast Peppers | Autumn Keto Pumpkin Bread | Chicharrones con Huevos (Pork Rind and Eggs) | Baked Buckwheat Pancakes with Hazelnuts |
| Glazed Sesame Ginger Salmon | Spicy Chicken Thighs | Blackberry and Grilled Chicken Salad | Sunday's Best Roast Beef |
| Lamb Cutlets with Garlic Sauce | Beanless Chili con Carne | Tomato Bredie | Pad Thai |

# Meat

## Portobello Mushroom Burgers

[Total Time: 25 MIN| Serve: 1]

*Ingredients:*

*½ tbsp coconut oil*

*1 tsp oregano*

*2 Portobello mushroom caps*

*1 garlic clove*

*Salt*

*Black pepper*

*1 tbsp Dijon mustard*

*¼ cup cheddar cheese*

*6 oz beef/bison*

Directions:

1. Heat a griddle and combine spices and oil in a bowl.

2. Remove gills from mushrooms and place into marinade until needed.

3. Add beef, cheese, salt, mustard, and pepper in another bowl and mix to combine; form into a patty.

4. Place marinated caps onto the grill and cook for 8 minutes until thoroughly heated. Place patty onto the grill and cook on each side for 5 minutes.

5. Take 'buns' from grill and top with burger and any other toppings you choose.

6. Serve.

   *[Calories 735 | Total Fats 48g | Net Carbs: 4g | Protein 60g | Fiber: 4g]*

# *Shrimp Stuffed Bell Peppers*

[Total Time: 2 HR 50 MIN| Serve: 3]

*Ingredients:*

*1 lb. shrimps, peeled and deveined*

*1 lb. ground pork*

*5 pcs bell peppers, chopped into quarters*

*4 pcs green onions, chopped*

*2 cloves of garlic, minced*

*1 organic egg*

*1 tbsp low-sodium soy sauce*

*1 tsp rice vinegar*

*2 tsp fish sauce*

*1 tsp five spice*

*Salt and pepper to taste*

*1 tbsp sesame oil*

Directions:

1. Add the spices, onions, sesame oil, fish sauce, and egg in a large Ziploc back.

2. Throw in the pork and shrimps in the bag and shake.

3. Place in the fridge to marinate for at least 2 hours.

4. Set the oven to 375 F when you're ready to cook.

5. Scoop the pork and shrimp mixture onto the bell pepper, place on a baking sheet and cook in the oven for 35 minutes.

6. Turn the tray around and then bake for another 5 minutes.

7. Allow to rest for 5 minutes before serving.

*[Calories 91 | Total Fats 4.7g | Net Carbs: 1.5g | Protein 9.9g | Fiber 12g]*

## Irish Styled Spiced Beef

[Total Time: 25 MIN| Serve: 4]

*Ingredients:*

*1 1/2 lbs. ground beef*

*½ cup red wine*

*2 cups mushrooms, sliced*

*1 bunch of broccoli, chopped into florets*

*2 cups baby spinach*

*3 tbsp keto Ketchup*

*2 tbsp low-sodium soy sauce*

*2 cloves of garlic, chopped*

*1 tsp cayenne*

*2 tsp cumin*

*½ tsp onion powder*

2 tsp ginger, minced

Salt and pepper to taste

Directions:

1.  Heat a cast iron skillet and add the ground beef. Brown the beef before adding the minced ginger and chopped garlic. Stir well.

2.  Add the broccoli to the pan as well as the spices and mix well.

3.  Pour the wine, along with the spinach and mushrooms. Stir and cook until the spinach has wilted.

4.  Add the keto Ketchup, stir, and serve hot.

    *[Calories 515 | Total Fats 35g | Net Carbs: 6g | Protein 33.25g | Fiber: 12g]*

## Beef Sirloin with Cilantro Sauce
[Total Time: 60 MIN| Serve: 3]

Ingredients:

1 lb. Sirloin tip cut

For the marinade:

¼ cup low-sodium soy sauce

4 tbsp lime juice

2 cloves of garlic minced

½ cup cilantro

¼ tsp chili pepper flakes

¼ cup olive oil

For the sauce:

¼ cup olive oil

2 cloves of garlic, minced

1 cup fresh cilantro

2 tbsp lemon juice

½ tsp coriander

½ tsp cumin

½ tsp salt

Directions:

1. Place all the ingredients for the marinade in a Ziploc bag. Add the beef, shake and then marinate in the fridge for at least 45 minutes.

2. Make the sauce while waiting for the beef to marinate. Add all the ingredients for the paste in a food processor and pulse until you achieve a smooth paste.

3. After marinating, sear the sirloin on a hot cast iron skillet heated over a medium-high fire.

4. Cook for 3-4 minutes on each side.

   [Calories 174 | Total Fats 18.7g | Net Carbs: 2.8g | Protein 32.2g | Fiber: 1g]

## Bacon wrapped Lasagna Twisted

[Total Time: 25 MIN| Serve: 2]

*Ingredients:*

*8 bacon strips*

*¼ cup all-natural pizza sauce*

*¼ lb. ground beef*

*1 cup mozzarella cheese, shredded*

*3 tbsp parmesan cheese, grated*

*1 tsp Italian seasoning*

Directions:

1.  Set oven to 350⁰F.

2.  In a pan, brown the beef over medium heat.

3.  Drain the fat from the beef when cooked and then sprinkle with the Italian seasoning.

4.  Layer 4 strips of bacon on a 9-inch baking dish and then spread half of the pizza sauce on top. Add the half of the ground beef and half of the mozzarella and parmesan and the cover with the remaining pcs. of bacon and repeat the process.

5.  Place in the oven to bake for 12-15 minutes or until the cheese has melted.

    *[Calories 702 | Total Fats 41g | Net Carbs: 10g | Protein 75g]*

## Macadamia-Crusted Lamb Chops with Ghee
[Total Time: 30 MIN| Serve: 2]

*Ingredients:*

*6 pcs lamb chops*

*¾ cup macadamia nuts, ground*

*2 tbsp fresh rosemary*

*Salt and pepper to taste*

*2 tbsp ghee*

Directions:

1. Set oven to 350⁰F.

2. Season the lamb chops with salt and pepper. Drizzle with ghee on top.

3. Combine the macadamia nuts and rosemary and roll the lamb chops in the mixture.

4. Place the lamb chops on a baking sheet lined with oil and place in the oven to cook for 25 minutes.

5. Serve warm.

*[Calories 856 | Total Fats 66g | Net Carbs: 9.1g | Protein 60.3g]*

## Roast Beef with Mushroom Soup
[Total Time: 6 HR 10 MIN| Serve: 4]

*Ingredients:*

*1.5 lb. beef roast*

*8oz cream of mushroom soup*

*½ tsp chili powder*

1 tsp smoked paprika

Salt and pepper to taste

Directions:

1.   Season the beef with chili powder, paprika, salt, and pepper.

2.   Place the beef in a slow cooker and pour over the mushroom soup.

3.   Cover and cook on low for 6 hours.

[Calories 252 | Total Fats 53.6g | Net Carbs: 6.4g | Protein 15g]

## Slow-Cooker Creamy Beef Stroganoff
[Total Time: 6 HR 10 MIN| Serve: 4]

Ingredients:

1 lb. beef, cut into cubes

16 oz. cream of mushroom soup

1 onion, chopped

2 carrots, sliced

1 pcs bay leaf

1 tbsp flour

2 tbsp ghee

Salt and pepper to taste

Directions:

1.   Season the beef with salt and pepper and then sprinkle with the flour.

2.  In a cast iron skillet, heat the ghee on medium fire and then add the beef until cooked through.
3.  Transfer the beef cubes in a slow cooker and then add the rest of the ingredients. Stir and then cover.
4.  Cook on low for 6 hours. Serve warm.

    *[Calories 345 | Total Fats 16.8g | Net Carbs: 10.8g | Protein 36.1g]*

## Mexican Meatballs

[Total Time: 35 MIN| Serve:6]

*Ingredients:*

*1 lb ground beef (92% lean)*

*4 oz white onion, minced*

*4 oz Monterey Jack cheese with spicy peppers*

*1 Tbsp butter*

*3 cloves garlic*

*1 tsp chili powder*

*1 tsp ground cumin*

*1 tsp ground coriander*

*1 egg*

*Sea salt and freshly ground pepper to taste*

Directions:

1.  Preheat oven to 350°F.
2.  In a frying pan, sauté onions in butter until translucent. Set aside

3. Shred and mince the Monterey Jack cheese with spicy peppers. Set aside.

4. In a mixing bowl, whisk the egg with ricotta cheese.

5. Add the spices, salt, and pepper and mix.

6. Add onions and minced Monterey Jack cheese with spicy peppers. Mix well.

7. Add beef and mix until all ingredients are combined.

8. Roll the meat mixture into a ball.

9. Place the meatballs on a cookie sheet, and bake about 20 minutes.

10. Serve hot.

*[Calories 321.28 | Total Fats 25.25g | Net Carbs: 2.94g | Protein 19.54g| Fibr 0.9g]*

## Ground Beef and Cheese Stuffed Bell Peppers
[Total Time: 30 MIN| Serve: 4]

*Ingredients:*

*1 lb Ground beef*

*2 Spring onions, sliced*

*1 tsp Ginger, diced*

*8 Eggs*

*2 Bell peppers, cut in half*

*2 tsp Garlic, diced*

*Salt*

*Black pepper*

*For Sauce:*

*1½ tbsp Rice wine vinegar*

*1 tbsp Chili Paste*

*1/3 cup Apricot preserves, sugar-free*

*1 tbsp Ketchup, low sugar*

*1 tbsp Soy sauce*

## Directions:

1. Season beef with pepper and salt and start cooking over a medium flame until browned. Add ginger and garlic and stir together.
2. Push beef to one side and put in spring onions, cook for 2 minutes then stir together with beef. Take from flame and put aside.
3. Add all sauce ingredients to a pan and cook for 3 minutes then add half to beef.
4. Stir sauce and beef together and use to stuff peppers.
5. Set oven to 350 F and bake for 15 minutes.
6. Top with reserved sauce and serve.
   *[Calories 470 | Total Fats 35g | Net Carbs: 6.3g | Protein 32.3g | Fiber: 5.3g]*

# Low Carb Burger

[Total Time: 60 MIN| Serve: 4]

*Ingredients:*

*1.1 lbs ground beef*

*1 small onion, finely chopped*

*1 red pepper, chopped*

*¼ cup cheese, grated*

*1 carrot, grated*

*1 baby marrow, grated*

*1 tsp ginger, grated*

*1 tsp crushed garlic*

*2 eggs*

*2 tbsp almond flour*

*1 tsp parsley, minced*

*1 tsp coriander*

*Salt and pepper to take*

Directions:

1.  Mix all ingredients together in a bowl.

2.  Form the mixture into balls and flatten into patties.

3.  Roll the patties in almond flour and leave to the firm in the fridge for around 30 minutes. This will help to keep the patties from falling apart while cooking.

4.  When firm, pan fry the patties in coconut oil. Make sure your oil is hot before adding patties to the pan,

you need to hear that oil sizzle. If the oil is not hot, the patty will stick to the pan and fall apart while cooking.

5.  Take 1 large brown mushroom, rub with olive oil and some crushed garlic, do not salt. And bake in the oven at 360⁰F for 15-20mins. Place the cooked burger on top of the mushroom, add grated cheese and melt in the oven for a couple of minutes.

6.  Add 1 tbsp. mayo to the finely diced red onion, lettuce and tomato, and place on top of the burger.

*[Calories 340    Total Fats 28g  |  Net Carbs: 3g  |  Protein 17g]*

## Meatballs in Fragrant Coconut Broth
[Total Time: 30 MIN| Serve: 4]

*Ingredients:*

*For meatballs:*

*1 lb. Ground beef*

*4 Garlic Cloves*

*2 Tbsp Almond milk*

*1 Tbsp Coconut oil*

*½ Onions*

*½ Cup Almond Flour*

*1 Tbsp Himalayan salt*

*For broth:*

*1 cup Broth of choice*

*1 Cup Coconut milk*

*Spices:*

*1 Tsp Turmeric*

*1 Tsp Crushed pepper (red)*

*Ginger*

*2 Tsp Coriander seeds*

*1 Tsp Cinnamon*

*1 Blade Lemongrass*

*Lime zest*

Directions:

1. Heat oil in a skillet and sauté garlic and onion until aromatic.

2. Mix together almond milk and flour to make a paste then add beef and salt.

3. Add onions and garlic to mixture and use hands to combine. Form into balls and put aside until needed.

4. Place meatballs in the skillet you used to sauté, arrange around the edge leaving the middle empty.

5. Add spices to the center of the pan while meatballs cook. When meatballs are browned all over pour in broth and coconut milk. Shake pan or gently stir to combine.

6. Add ginger and lemongrass and cook for 15 minutes.

7. Check if meatballs are cooked, if not cook for an additional 5 minutes.

8.  Serve.

> *[Calories 566 | Total Fats 38g | Net Carbs: 4g | Protein 24g | Fiber: 2g]*

## *Baked Pork Chops with Apple, Rosemary*
[Total Time: 20 MIN| Serve: 2]

*Ingredients:*

*For Pork Chops:*

*2 Tbsp Olive oil*

*Black pepper*

*½ Apple*

*4 Pork Chops*

*Salt to taste*

*Paprika*

*4 Rosemary Sprigs*

*For Vinaigrette:*

*1 Tbsp Lemon juice*

*Salt to taste*

*2 Tbsp olive oil*

*2 Tbsp apple cider vinegar*

*1 Tbsp maple syrup (sugar-free)*

*Black pepper*

Directions:

1.  Set oven to 400⁰F and place cast iron skillet into the oven to be heated.

2. Dry pork chops and season with oil, paprika, pepper, and salt.

3. Place pork into skillet and sear for 2 minutes per side over a high flame.

4. Add rosemary and apple to pork and bake for 10 minutes until pork is thoroughly cooked.

5. Combine all ingredients for vinaigrette except oil then add oil before serving.

6. Serve.

*[Calories 485 | Total Fats 41.2g | Net Carbs: 4g | Protein 25g | Fiber: 1g]*

## *Lemon-Mustard Pork Chops*

[Total Time: 20 MIN| Serve: 2]

*Ingredients:*

*For Pork:*

*1 Tbsp Salt*

*1 Tsp Paprika*

*16 oz. Pork loins (4)*

*1 Tsp Black pepper*

*1 Tsp Thyme*

*For Mustard Sauce:*

*¼ cup Heavy Cream*

*½ Lemons*

*½ cup Chicken Broth*

*1 Tsp Apple cider Vinegar*

*1 Tbsp mustard*

Directions:

1. Rinse pork loin and use paper towels to pat dry. Season with salt, thyme, paprika, and pepper.
2. Heat a skillet and sear pork for 3 minutes per side.
3. Remove from skillet and put aside.
4. Use vinegar and broth to deglaze the pan. Add cream and stir to combine.
4. Add mustard and squeeze lemon juice into sauce. Return pork to pot and use the sauce to coat.
5. Cook for 10 minutes until pork is thoroughly cooked.
6. Serve with the desired side.

   *[Calories 480 | Total Fats 30g | Net Carbs: 1g | Protein 46g | Fiber 1g]*

## *Loaded Cauliflower and Bacon Casserole*
[Total Time: 1 HR 40 MIN| Serve: 6]

*Ingredients:*

*For Beef:*

*1 tbsp Bacon fat*

*1 tsp Cumin*

*½ tsp Chili powder*

*¼ tsp Cayenne pepper*

*¼ tsp Black pepper*

1 tbsp Ketchup, low sugar

1 tsp Fish sauce

1 lb Ground beef

2 tsp Garlic

½ tsp Paprika

½ tsp Salt

¼ tsp Onion powder

¼ tsp Mrs. Dash seasoning

1 tbsp Soy sauce

For Casserole:

1 Cauliflower head, florets

4 oz Cheddar cheese

10 oz Bacon, fried and chopped

4 oz Cream cheese

Directions:

1.  Add all ingredients for ground beef to a bowl except fish sauce, soy sauce, and ketchup. Use hands to combine then add to a plastic bag and add fish sauce, soy sauce, and ketchup.

2.  Rub together in bag and seal; place into refrigerator for 30 minutes or more.

3.  Cook bacon until crisp, remove from pot and chop; save grease for use later.

4.  Add beef to grease in a pot and cook until browned all over.

5. Layer cauliflower in a baking dish and top with cooked beef and cream cheese then add bacon and top with cheddar cheese.

6. Set oven to 350⁰F. Bake for 50 minutes until golden and cheese has melted.

7. Serve.

   *[Calories 575 | Total Fats 46.3g | Net Carbs: 4.4g | Protein 26.8g | Fiber 2.2g]*

## Roasted Poblano Stuffed with Pork

[Total Time: 30 MIN| Serve: 4]

*Ingredients:*

*1 tbsp Bacon fat*

*½ Onion, chopped*

*7 Baby mushrooms, chopped*

*1 tsp Cumin*

*Salt*

*1 lb Ground Pork*

*4 Poblano peppers*

*1 Vine tomato*

*¼ cup Cilantro*

*1 tsp Chili powder*

*Black pepper*

Directions:

1. Slice peppers and remove seeds, place peppers onto a baking sheet lined with foil and broil for 10 minutes. Turn every 2 minutes so as to cook evenly.

2. Heat bacon fat in a skillet and cook pork for 10 minutes. Add pepper, chili, salt, and cumin to pork, stir to combine.

3. Add garlic and onion, cook, until soft then add mushrooms.

4. Add tomatoes and cilantro to the pan and cook for 2 minutes.

5. Set oven to 350⁰F. Uses pork mixtures to fill peppers.

6. Bake for 8 minutes.

7. Serve warm.

*[Calories 367 | Total Fats 27.3g | Net Carbs: 5g | Protein 21.3g | Fiber: 2.3g]*

## *Ultra-Crispy Skin Slow Roasted Pork Shoulder*
[Total Time: 12 HR| Serve: 20]

*Ingredients:*

*3 ½ tbsp Salt*

*1 tsp Black pepper*

*1 tsp Onion powder*

*8 lbs Pork shoulder*

*2 tsp Oregano*

*1 tsp Onion powder*

Directions:

1.  Rinse and dry pork and let it sit at room temperature for a few hours.

2.  Set oven to 250⁰F. Combine seasonings and rub pork all over.

3.  Line baking sheet with foil and place a wire rack onto sheets, bake for 10 hours and remove from oven.

4.  Cover with foil and put aside for 15 minutes. Set oven to 500⁰F and return pork to oven without foil. Bake for 20 minutes, turning every 5 minutes.

5.  Remove from oven, cover with foil and let it sit for 20 minutes.

6.  Slice and serve.

    *[Calories 461 | Total Fats 36.7g | Net Carbs: 0.2g | Protein 30.3g | Fiber: 0.1g]*

## *Italian-Style Meatballs*

[Total Time: 25 MIN| Serve: 4]

*Ingredients:*

*1 tsp Oregano*

*2 tsp Garlic, diced*

*3 tbsp Tomato paste*

*2 Eggs*

*½ cup Mozzarella cheese*

Salt

1 ½ lbs Ground beef

½ tsp Italian seasoning

½ tsp Onion powder

3 tbsp Flaxseed meal

½ cup Olives, sliced

1 tsp Worcestershire sauce

Black pepper

Directions:

1. Set oven to 400⁰F.

2. Add beef to a bowl along with Italian seasoning, onion powder, flaxseed meal, olives, Worcestershire sauce, oregano, garlic, tomato paste, eggs, mozzarella cheese, pepper, and salt.

3. Mix together and form into balls and place onto a baking sheet lined with foil.

4. Bake for 20 minutes.

5. Serve.

   *[Calories 594 | Total Fats 44.8g | Net Carbs: 3.8g | Protein 36.8g | Fiber: 2.3g]*

## Korean-Style Grilled Short Ribs
[Total Time: 2 HR 15 MIN| Serve: 4]

*Ingredients:*

*For marinade and ribs:*

¼ cup Soy sauce

2 tbsp Fish sauce

1 ½ lbs Short rib

2 tbsp Rice vinegar

For spice rub:

½ tsp Onion powder

½ tsp Red pepper flakes

¼ tsp Cardamom

1 tsp Ground ginger

½ tsp Garlic, diced

½ tsp Sesame seed

1 tbsp Salt

Directions:

1. Combine all ingredients for marinade in a bowl and place ribs into marinade; put aside for 1-2 hours.

2. Transfer ribs and marinade into a baking dish. Combine spice rub and coat ribs all over.

3. Heat grill and cook for 10 minutes. Alternately you may place ribs into a grill pan and place into oven for 15 minutes.

4. Serve warm.

*[Calories 417 | Total Fats 31.8g | Net Carbs: 0.9g | Protein 29.5g]*

## Bacon Cheeseburger Waffles

[Total Time: 30 MIN| Serve: 4]

*Ingredients:*

*For Waffles:*

*2 Eggs*

*¼ tsp Garlic powder*

*4 tbsp Almond Flour*

*Salt*

*1.5 oz Cheddar cheese*

*1 cup Cauliflower, crumbled*

*¼ tsp Onion powder*

*3 tbsp Parmesan cheese*

*Black pepper*

*For topping:*

*4 Bacon slices, chopped*

*1.5 oz Cheddar cheese, shredded*

*4 oz Ground beef*

*4 tbsp BBQ sauce, sugar-free*

*Salt*

*Black pepper*

## Directions:

1. Add crumbled cauliflower to a bowl along with parmesan, spices, almond flour, half of cheddar cheese and eggs.

2.   Heat skillet and cook bacon for 2 minutes then add beef and cook thoroughly. Transfer any grease from meats into cauliflower mix.

3.   Blend the waffle mixture with an immersion blender.

4.   Heat waffle iron and pour in mixture.

5.   Add bbq sauce to meat as waffles cook.

6.   Transfer waffles to a plate and top with cheese; broil for 2 minutes.

7.   Serve.

*[Calories 354 | Total Fats 29.8g | Net Carbs: 3g | Protein 18.8g | Fiber: 1.5g]*

## Classic Pan-Seared Ribeye Steak

[Total Time: 20 MIN| Serve: 3]

*Ingredients:*

*2 medium Ribeye steaks*

*Salt*

*Black pepper*

*3 tbsp Bacon fat*

Directions:

1.   Set oven to $250^0$F.

2.   Place a wire rack on a baking sheet and place steaks on the rack.

3.   Use pepper and salt to season steaks and bake until steak's internal temperature is $123^0$F.

4.  Melt fat in a cast iron pan until it is extremely hot then transfer steaks to pot and sear on both sides.

5.  Let steaks sit for a few minutes before slicing.

6.  Serve.

    *[Calories 430 | Total Fats 31.7g | Net Carbs: 0g | Protein 30.3g | Fiber: 0g]*

## *Herb Roasted Beef Slow Cooker*
[Total Time: 8 HR 10 MIN| Serve: 5]

*Ingredients:*

*1 ½ lbs. lean beef*

*2 celery ribs*

*1 cup beef broth*

*2 Tbsp amaranth flour*

*2 Tbsp almond butter*

*2 Tbsp olive oil*

*1 tsp mustard*

*2 Tbsp fresh lemon juice*

*4 Tbsp chopped parsley*

*Salt, pepper,vdried thyme, dried marjoram*

Directions:

1.  In a bowl, toss the beef with the amaranth flour. Heat the butter and oil in a skillet; add the beef and cook, stirring, until browned.

2.  In a slow cooker combine the browned beef with remaining ingredients, except lemon juice and parsley.

3.  Cover and cook on LOW for 6 to 8 hours.

4.  Once ready, stir in lemon juice and parsley and serve hot.

    *[Calories 387.96 | Total Fats 12.53g | Net Carbs: 2.56g | Protein 20.96g | Fiber: 0.02g]*

## *Lamb Chop with Garlic Sauce*

[Total Time: 40 MIN| Serve: 10]

*Ingredients:*

*4 lbs. lamb cutlets*

*1 small head of garlic, cloves peeled*

*2 Tbsp apple cider vinegar*

*½ cup water*

*1/4 cup extra-virgin olive oil*

*Pinch salt and black ground pepper to taste*

Directions:

1.  Crush the garlic cloves thoroughly in a mortar. In a bowl, add the vinegar and water and mix it well with the crushed garlic. Set aside.

2.  In a large frying pan, pour the olive oil and fry the lamb cutlets until nicely brown.

3.  Add the garlic mixture and let it cook gently for about 10 minutes.

4.  Shake the frying pan to spread the garlic mixture evenly over the lamb.

5.  Season with salt and black pepper to taste. Serve.

    *[Calories 416 | Total Fats 28g | Net Carbs: 0.16g | Protein 36g | Fiber: 0.1g]*


## Mexican Style Meatballs

[Total Time: 35 MIN| Serve: 6]

*Ingredients:*

*1 lb. ground beef (92% lean)*

*4 oz. white onion, minced*

*4 oz. Monterey Jack cheese with spicy peppers*

*1 Tbsp butter*

*3 cloves garlic*

*1 1 tsp chili powder*

*1 tsp ground cumin*

*1 tsp ground coriander*

*1 egg*

*Sea salt and freshly ground pepper to taste*

Directions:

1.  Preheat oven to 350⁰F.

2.  In a frying pan, sauté onions in butter until translucent. Set aside

3. Shred and mince the Monterey Jack cheese with spicy peppers. Set aside.
4. In a mixing bowl, whisk the egg with ricotta cheese. Add the spices, salt, and pepper and mix.
5. Add onions and minced Monterey Jack cheese with spicy peppers. Mix well.
6. Add beef and mix until all ingredients are combined.
7. Roll the meat mixture into a ball.
8. Place the meatballs on a cookie sheet, and bake about 20 minutes.
9. Serve hot.

*[Calories 321 | Total Fats 25g | Net Carbs: 2.9g | Protein 19g | Fiber: 0.9g]*

## *Oven-Baked Meatballs Cheesy Sauce*
[Total Time: 35 MIN| Serve: 6]

*Ingredients:*

*1 lb. ground beef (lean)*

*2 white onion*

*1 cup grated Cheddar cheese*

*4 oz. Gruyere cheese*

*1 egg*

*1.5 tsp nutmeg*

*1.5 tsp allspice*

*Sea salt and freshly black pepper to taste*

*Butter for greasing*

Directions:

1.  Preheat oven to 350⁰F.

2.  In a greased frying pan, sauté onions until translucent. Remove from heat, and let cool.

3.  In a food processor mince the Gruyere cheese. Set aside.

4.  In a mixing bowl, whisk the egg with grated Cheddar cheese. Add the spices, salt, and pepper and mix.

5.  Add in onions and Gruyere cheese. Mix well until smooth.

6.  Add the beef and mix until all ingredients are combined well.

7.  Divide meat mixture and roll each piece into a ball.

8.  Place the meatballs on a cookie sheet, and bake in preheated oven about 20 minutes. Serve hot.

    *[Calories 385 | Total Fats 29g | Net Carbs: 4.7g | Protein 25g | Fiber 0.9g]*


## *Sticky-Asian Short Ribs*

[Total Time: 20 MIN| Serve: 3]

*Ingredients:*

*1 ½ lb. short ribs*

*For the rub:*

*1 tsp ginger, grated*

*1 clove of garlic, minced*

*½ tsp onion powder*

*½ tsp red pepper flakes*

*¼ tsp cardamom*

*½ tsp sesame seed*

*1 tsp salt*

*For the marinade:*

*¼ low-sodium soy sauce*

*2 tbsp fish sauce*

*2 tbsp rice vinegar*

Directions:

1.  Whisk all the ingredients for the marinade and pour it over the ribs. Allow the ribs to marinate for an hour.

2.  Mix all the ingredients for the rubbing.

3.  Roll marinated ribs in the rubbing and making sure to evenly coat.

4.  Heat the grill and cook for 4-5 minutes on each side.

    *[Calories 417 | Total Fats 31.8g | Net Carbs: 0.9g | Protein 29.5g]*

## Beanless Low Carb Chili Con Carne

[Total Time: 60 MIN| Serve: 5]

*Ingredients:*

*1 lb Ground beef*

*1 Greenvpepper, chopped*

*1 Onion, chopped*

2 tbsp Curry powder

2 tbsp Cumin

1 tbsp Coconut oil

1 tsp Onion powder

1 tsp Black pepper

1 lb Italian sausage, spicy

1 Yellow pepper, chopped

16 oz Tomato sauce

2 tbsp Chili powder

1 tbsp Garlic, diced

1 tbsp Butter

1 tsp Salt

Directions:

1. Heat oil and butter in a pan, heat thoroughly and add garlic, onions and bell peppers. Cook for 3 minutes then add beef and sausage.

2. Cook for 5 minutes until browned then add onion and chili powder. Stir to combine and add tomato sauce. Lower flame and cook for 20ominutes.

3. Add cumin and curry, stir and cook for 45ominutes or until chili thickens to your liking.

   *[Calories 415 | Total Fats 25g | Net Carbs: 6g |* **Protein 146g** *| Fiber 51]*

# Classic Beef Meatloaf

[Total Time: 1 HR 20 MIN| Serve: 4]

*Ingredients:*

*7 oz prosciutto, sliced thin*

*7 oz provolone, sliced thin*

*2 cups baby spinach*

*1 cup tomato sauce*

*½ cup tomato paste*

*1 tbsp apple cider vinegar*

*4 tbsp stevia*

*1 lb. ground pork*

*½ onion, chopped*

*½ cup bell pepper, chopped*

*2 cloves of garlic, minced*

*¼ cup parmesan cheese, grated*

*2 organic eggs*

*1 tsp oregano, dried*

*1 tsp basil, dried*

*Salt and pepper to taste*

*1 tbsp butter*

Directions:

1. Set the oven at 350⁰F.

2. Melt the butter in a pan over medium fire. Throw in the baby spinach and season with salt and pepper. Cook until the leaves wilt.

3.  In a bowl combine the tomato sauce and paste, along with the apple cider and stevia. Stir and set aside.

4.  In another bowl, combine the pork, onion, bell pepper, garlic, parmesan, and herbs. Mix well.

5.  Lay a parchment paper about 10 inches and spread the meat on top. Arrange the prosciutto on top followed by the spinach and provolone to create a meatloaf. Seal sides.

6.  Place the meatloaf in a loaf panolined with foil and pour the tomato sauce on top.

7.  Bake in the oven for a little over an hour or until the inner temperature reaches 165$^0$F.

*[Calories 516 | Total Fats 37g | Net Carbs: 8g | Protein 37g]*


## *Oven Roasted Pulled Pork Shoulder*
[Total Time: 5 HR 10 MIN| Serve: 4]

*Ingredients:*

*2 lbs. whole pork shoulder*

*2 tsp paprika*

*1 tsp salt*

*1 tsp pepper*

*½ tsp cumin*

*¼ tsp cinnamon*

Directions:

1. Set the oven at 450⁰F.

2. Score the skin of the pork with a sharp knife.

3. Combine all of the ingredients of the rub and then smother it over the pork.

4. Place in a baking dish and cook in the oven for 30 mins.

5. Take off from the oven and cover the dish with a foil.

6. Lower the heat to 350 F and place the covered dish in the oven to cook for another 4 hours and 30 mins.

7. Take the pork out of the oven and pull using forks. Serve with a low-carb BBQ sauce.

    *[Calories 534 | Total Fats 39g | Net Carbs: 0.9g | Protein 42.4g | Fiber: 0.5g]*

## Greek Slow Roasted Lamb

[Total Time: 7 HR 15 MIN| Serve: 3]

*Ingredients:*

*1 lb. leg of lamb*

*2 tbsp Dijon mustard*

*3 cloves of garlic*

*3 sprigs of thyme*

*½ tsp rosemary, dried*

*3 pcs mint leaves*

*1 tbsp liquid stevia*

¼ *cup olive oil*

*Salt and pepper to taste*

Directions:

1.  Cut large slits on the leg of lamb and place in a slow cooker.

2.  Combine the mustard, olive oil and stevia and then rub over the lamb. Season with salt and pepper.

3.  Inset the garlic and rosemary of the slits.

4.  Cover and cook on low for 7 hours.

5.  Add the mint leaves and thyme after 7 hours and cook for another hour.

*[Calories 413 | Total Fats 35.2g | Net Carbs: 0.5g | Protein 26g]*

## *Lamb and Spinach Curry*

[Total Time: 8 HR 25 MIN| Serve: 5]

*Ingredients:*

*1/3 cup Coconut or olive oil*

*3 chopped yellow onions*

*4 cloves garlic, peeled and minced*

*2cm piece of ginger, peeled and grated*

*2 tsp Ground cumin*

*1 ½ tsp Cayenne pepper*

*1½ tsp Ground turmeric*

*2 cups Beef stock, high quality*

*53 oz Leg of lamb cut into 2cm cubes*

*Salt*

*6 cups Baby spinach*

*1 1/5 cups Plain full-fat yogurt*

Directions:

1. Place oil into a large skillet over medium to high heat.

2. Add chopped onions and garlic into the skillet and sauté until brown, 4 - 5 minutes.

3. Then add ginger, cayenne pepper, turmeric, and cumin to the skillet. Stir and let the flavor develop for 30 seconds.

4. Pour in beef stock and scrape the browned bits off the bottom of the skillet.

5. Once the stock comes to a boil, take the skillet off the heat.

6. Place the lamb in your slow cooker. Add the contents of skillet and 1 tbsp of salt.

7. Cover the slow cooker with the lid and cook on high for 4 hours or low for 8 hours. 5 minutes before the slow cooker is done, stir the spinach into the dish wait for it to wilt.

8. Before serving, stir in the yogurt.

9. Serve and enjoy.

*[Calories 304 | Total Fats 16.32g | Net Carbs: 5.5g | Protein 32.85g]*


## Cheeseburger Casserole

[Total Time: 45 MIN| Serve: 6]

*Ingredients:*

*3 Bacon slices*

*1 ¼ cups Cauliflower*

*½ tsp Garlic powder*

*2 tbsp Ketchup, no sugar*

*2 tbsp Mayonnaise*

*4 oz Cheddar cheese*

*1 lb Ground beef*

*½ cup Almond Flour*

*1 tbsp Psyllium Husk Powder*

*½ tsp Onion powder*

*1 tbsp Dijon mustard*

*3 Eggs*

*Salt*

*Black pepper*

Directions:

1.  Set oven to 350⁰F.

2.  Place cauliflower into a processor and pulse until fine like rice. Add remaining dry ingredients except for cheese.

3. Add beef and bacon in processor until combined and pasty.

4. Heat skillet and cook meat for 8 minutes then add to dry ingredients in a bowl along with half of cheese. Stir to combine and line a baking dish with parchment paper.

5. Press mixture into dish and top with left over cheese.

6. Bake for 30 minutes on top rack.

7. Take from heat, cool and slice.

8. Serve.

   *[Calories 478 | Total Fats 35.5g | Net Carbs: 3.6g | Protein 32.2g | Fiber 3.3g]*

## *Leftover Teriyaki Beef Salad*

[Total Time: 10 MIN| Serve: 1]

*Ingredients:*

*1 cup left-over meat (chicken or pork), shredded*

*2 cups iceberg lettuce*

*1 tbsp mayonnaise*

*2 tbsp sour cream*

*Salt and pepper to taste*

Directions:

1. Whisk the mayo and sour cream in a salad bowl.

2. Add the lettuce to the bowl along with the shredded meat.
3. Season with salt and pepper and toss.
4. Serve immediately.

   *[Calories 252 | Total Fats 53.6g | Net Carbs: 6.4g | Protein 15g | Fiber: 1.2g]*


## Grilled Asian-Flavored Steak

[Total Time: 55 MIN| Serve: 4]

*Ingredients:*

*4 pcs steak*

*For the glaze marinade:*

*½ tsp sesame oil*

*½ tsp chili flakes*

*1 tsp ginger, grated*

*½ cup low-sodium soy sauce*

*2 pcs green onions*

Directions:

1. Combine all the ingredients for the marinade in a large bowl and whisk well.
2. Place the steaks in the bowl and marinate for at least 45 minutes.
3. Heat the grill on high and cook the steaks for 5 minutes on each side, or depending on your liking.

*[Calories 531 | Total Fats 13.7g | Net Carbs: 4.7g | Protein 94.4g]*

# Quick Stir-Fry Beef

[Total Time: 25 MIN| Serve: 2]

*Ingredients:*

*1 tbsp olive oil*

*12 oz sirloin steak, cut into strips*

*1 onion, chopped*

*2 cloves of garlic, crushed*

*1 cup cherry tomatoes, quartered*

*1 red bell pepper chopped*

*2 tsp ginger, grated*

*4 tbsp organic apple cider vinegar*

*Salt and pepper to taste*

Directions:

1. Drizzle the olive oil on a non-stick pan and heat over medium fire.

2. Season the sirloin with salt and pepper and sear in the hot oil for 4 minutes on each side.

3. While waiting, whisk the ginger and apple cider together and pour over the steak in the pan.

4. Add the chopped onion, garlic, bell pepper, and cherry tomatoes with the beef and reduce the fire to low.

5.  Cover the pan and allow to simmer for 5 minutes.

6.  Turn off the heat and then allow the beef to rest for 5 minutes before serving.

    *[Calories 359 | Total Fats 19g | Net Carbs: 10g | Protein 39]*


## Pizza Lettuce Wrap

[Total Time: 15 MIN| Serve: 2]

*Ingredients:*

*6 pcs Romaine lettuce leaves*

*3 tbsp mayonnaise*

*6 slices of provolone cheese*

*6 slices salami*

*6 slices pepperoni*

*6 slice ham*


Directions:

1.  Lay the lettuce leaves on a serving plate.

2.  Spread the mayonnaise on top of the leaves and layer with the cheese, salami, pepperoni, and ham.

3.  Carefully roll the leaves and secure with a toothpick.

4.  Serve and immediately.

    *[Calories 592 | Total Fats 46g | Net Carbs: 6g | Protein 37g | Fiber: 1.1g]*

## Cheese Stuffed Bacon Wrapped Hot Dogs

[Total Time: 15 MIN| Serve: 2]

*Ingredients:*

*1 tbsp ghee*

*1 onion, chopped*

*1 red bell pepper, chopped*

*1 pc jalapeno, seeds removed and chopped*

*4 pcs beef hot dogs*

*4 bacon strips*

*3 cheddar cheese slices*

Directions:

1.  Heat the ghee in a non-stick pan over medium fire.

2.  Add the onions, bell peppers, and chopped jalapeno and sauté for 4 minutes. Remove from the pan and set aside

3.  Wrap the hotdog with bacon strips and secure with a toothpick. And cook in the same pan where the peppers were cooked.

4.  Fry the dogs for 5 minutes or until crispy on both sides.

5.  Lay the cheese slices on top of the cooking hotdogs and cover for 30 seconds to cook, or until the cheese melts.

6.  Serve the hot dogs with the sautéed peppers on the side.

*[Calories 349 | Total Fats 29g | Net Carbs: 8g | Protein 14g]*

## Savoury Mince

[Total Time: 25 MIN| Serve: 10]

*Ingredients:*

*4 tbsp coconut oil*

*2.2 lbs beef*

*2 onions finely diced*

*4 cups mixed Vegetables*

*4 carrots finely grated*

*1 packet gluten-free gravy*

*½ cup tomato paste*

*1 cup chicken stock*

Directions:

1.  Heat coconut oil in a pan and fry chopped onion, beef mince with and tomato paste and fry.
2.  Add chopped vegetables and grated carrot to the cooked mince.
3.  Continue to cook on a low heat until the vegetables are well cooked.
4.  If your mixture seems to be drying out, keep adding chicken stock to keep at the right consistency.

5. The longer you cook this mixture, the more the flavors will infuse through the mince.

6. Add gluten-free gravy.

   *[Calories 298 | Total Fats 12.1g | Net Carbs: 14g | Protein 32.7g | Fiber: 5.3g]*

## *Spring Roll in a Bowl*
[Total Time: 25 MIN| Serve: 12]

*Ingredients:*

*1.1 lbs pork mince*

*2 cups cabbage, shredded finely*

*2 cup grated carrot*

*2 cups grated baby marrows*

*1 cup mushrooms*

*4 tbsp coconut oil*

*1/2 cup soya sauce*

*1 cup chicken stock*

*2 tsp vinegar*

*5 cloves garlic, minced*

*4 tsp grated ginger*

*4 finely sliced spring onions*

*½ cup toasted sesame seeds*

*1 hard-boiled egg, chopped*

Directions:

1. Heat the coconut oil and fry the garlic, spring onions, ginger.

2. Add the pork mince and brown.

3. Add the cabbage and carrot to the pot and toss to combine. Stir in the soy sauce.

4. Cover and cook until the vegetables are soft, about 15 minutes.

5. Dish up, add chopped hard-boiled egg over each of the bowls.

6. Garnish with sesame seeds once you have dished up.

*[Calories 219 | Total Fats 9.7g | Net Carbs: 32.6g | Protein 3.2g]*

## Homemade Meatballs
[Total Time: 25 MIN| Serve: 12]

*Ingredients:*

*1.1 lbs ground beef*

*1 whole egg*

*½ cup almond flour*

*2 cloves of garlic, minced*

*1 tsp oregano, dried*

*1 tsp thyme, dried*

*1 cup mozzarella cheese, shredded*

*Saltvand pepper to taste*

*½ cup homemade marinara sauce*

Directions:

1. Preheat oven to 450⁰F.

2. In a large bowl, place the ground beef, egg, almond flour, garlic, oregano, thyme, and season with salt and pepper. Also, add the cheese.

3. Using your hands, mix all the ingredientsvtogether; making sure that everything is well combined.

4. Create 25 pcs of meatballs and lay them on a baking sheet lined with parchment paper.

5. Cook in the oven to cook for 15 minutes or until golden brown.

6. Serve the meatballs with marinara sauce.

   *[Calories 117 | Total Fats 9.3g | Net Carbs: 0.9g | Protein 7g]*

# Shredded Beef Salad
[Total Time: 10 MIN| Serve: 2]

*Ingredients:*

*2 cups beef, shredded*

*1 yellow pepper, sliced thinly lengthwise*

*1 white onion, sliced lengthwise*

*6 butter lettuce*

*2 tsp mayo*

*1/8 tsp chili flakes*

Directions:

1. Place the butter lettuce on a serving plate. Spread mayo on the lettuce and top with the shredded beef.

2. Place pepper slices and onions on top and season with chili flakes.

3. Serve as it is or rolled.

   [Calories 338 | Total Fats 25g | Net Carbs: 2.4g | Protein 24g]

## Crescent Roll Hotdog Pockets

[Total Time: 50 MIN| Serve: 2]

*Ingredients:*

*2 beef hot dogs*

*2 thick sticks of quick-melt cheese (or mozzarella)*

*4 slices of bacon*

*1/8 tsp garlic powder*

*1/8 tsp onion powder*

*Salt and pepper to taste*

Directions:

1. Preheat oven to 400⁰F.

2. Cut the hotdogs lengthwise to create slits.

3. Insert the cheese sticks in the hotdog and then wrap the bacon around the beef hot dog. Secure the bacon using a toothpick.

4. Transfer the hotdogs on a baking sheet lined with foil and flavor with garlic and onion powder.

5. Place in the oven to cook for 40 minutes or until the hotdogs turns golden brown and the cheese is melted.

6. Serve with a veggie salad on the side.

*[Calories 378 | Total Fats 35g | Net Carbs: 0.3g | Protein 17g]*

## Low-Carb Cheese Steak Salad

[Total Time: 35 MIN| Serve: 2]

*Ingredients:*

*For steaks:*

*¼ Tsp Salt*

*2 Tbsp Ghee*

*10.6 oz Ribeye steak*

*For salad:*

*2 ½ oz onionsv(sliced)*

*1 Green pepper (sliced)*

*½ Cup Cheddar cheese (grated)*

*Salt*

*1 Tbsp Ghee*

*1 Garlicvclove (diced)*

*1 Red pepper (sliced)*

*7 oz. Mixed greens*

*Fresh herbs*

Directions:

1.  Let steaks sit at room temperature for 15 minutes. Pat dry with paper towel and melt ghee. Coat with ghee, pepper, and salt.

2.  Heat a cast iron pot and sear steaks for 4 minutes until browned all over. Lower heat and cook steak until desired doneness have been achieved.

3.  Take steaks from pots and put aside to rest for 7 minutes then slice.

4.  Slice vegetables and add ghee to skillet and melt. Cook for 5 minutes until veggies are crisp.

5.  Add lettuce to bowl and top with cooked veggies, steak, and top with cheese.

6.  Serve warm.

    *[Calories 622 | Total Fats 47.1g | Net Carbs: 12.3g | Protein 38.1g | Fiber 4g]*

## Sausage and Cheese Balls

[Total Time: 20 MIN| Serve: 12]

*Ingredients:*

*12 Cubes Cheddar cheese*

*6 oz. Cheddar cheese (shredded)*

*12 oz. Ground sausage*

Directions:

1.  Combine sausage and cheese in a bowl.

2. Divide mixture into 12 parts.

3. Place cheese in middle of sausage mixture and form into balls.

4. Place on a try and put into the freezer.

5. Heat oil in a deep pot and fry for 5 minutes.

6. Serve warm.

   *[Calories 173 | Total Fats 14g | Net Carbs: 1g | Protein 10g | Fiber: 0g]*


## Almond Butter Bastie Bunless Bacon Burger

[Total Time: 50 MIN| Serve: 4]

*Ingredients:*

*For Almond Sauce:*

*1 cup water*

*4 Thai chilis*

*1 tsp swerve*

*1 cup almond butter*

*4 garlicvcloves*

*6 tbsp coconut amino*

*1 tbsp rice vinegar*

*For Burger:*

*4 pepper jack cheese slices*

*1 red onion, sliced*

*Salt*

*1 ½ lbs ground beef*

*8 baconvslices*

*8 romaine lettuce leaves*

*Black pepper*

Directions:

1. Prepare almond butter sauce by adding water and almond butter to a saucepan.
2. Heat mixture until it starts to thicken, stirring occasionally then add coconut aminos.
3. Add garlic, vinegar, Swerve and peppers, pulse until thoroughly combined.
4. Transfer pepper mixture to butter sauce in pot and mix together.
5. Put aside until needed.
6. Prepare burgers by seasoning beef with pepper and salt. Shape into patties and make an indent in each.
7. Place patties on baking sheet and put into the broiler for 7 minutes until golden. Flip patties and broil for an additional 7 minutes.
8. Top with cheese and bake for 5 minutes until melted.
9. Slice onionsvand cook bacon.
10. Arrange burgers by placing patties onto lettuce and topping with almond sauce, onion and bacon.
11. Serve.

*[Calories 890 | Total Fats 68g | Net Carbs: 8g | Protein 54.4g | Fiber: 10g]*

## Pigs in a Blanket

[Total Time: 40 MIN| Serve: 36]

*Ingredients:*

*8 oz cheddar cheese*

*1 tbsp Psyllium Husk powder*

*1 egg*

*½ tsp black pepper*

*37 mini hot dogs*

*3/ cup almond flour*

*3 tbsp cream cheese*

*½ tsp salt*

*½ tsp black pepper*

Directions:

1. Place mozzarella in a microwave safe dish and heat until cheese melts and is bubbling.

2. Add flour, salt, pepper and husk powder to cheese and mix together until dough is formed.

3. Spread dough on a plate and place into refrigerator for 20 minutes until firm.

4. Set oven to 400⁰F.

5. Transfer chilled dough to a piece of foilvand slice into 37 strips.

6.  Wrap each hot dog and place onto baking sheet. Bake for 15 minutes and broil for 2 minutes.

7.  Serve warm.

    *[Calories 72 | Total Fats 5.9g | Net Carbs: 0.6g | Protein 3.8g |Fiber: 0.4g]*


## Cheese Stuffed Bacon wrapped Hot Dogs
[Total Time: 45 MIN| Serve: 6]

*Ingredients:*

*6 Hot dogs*

*2 oz cheddar cheese*

*½ tsp onion powder*

*12 bacon slices*

*½ tsp garlic powder*

*Salt*

*Black pepper*

Directions:

1.  Set oven to 400⁰F.

2.  Slice each hot dog open and fill with cheese slices.

3.  Use 2 slices of bacon to wrap each hot dog and use toothpicks to hold in place.

4.  Place a wire rack on top of a baking sheet and add wrapped hot dogs. Season with garlic and onion powder.

5.  Bake for 40 minutes.

6. Serve warm.

*[Calories 380 | Total Fats 34.5g | Net Carbs: 0.3g | Protein 16.8g]*

## Cheesy Crust Pizza

[Total Time: 35 MIN| Serve: 12]

*Ingredients:*

*½ lb ground beef*

*2 eggs*

*1 tsp garlic powder*

*¼ tsp basil*

*¼ tsp turmeric*

*8 oz cream cheese*

*1 chorizo sausage*

*¼ cup parmesan cheese, grated*

*½ tsp cumin*

*½ tsp Italian seasoning*

*Salt*

*Black pepper*

Directions:

1. Set oven to 375⁰F.

2. Add parmesan cheese, pepper, garlic, cream cheese and eggs to a bowl and use a hand mixer to combine until smooth.

3.  Coat baking pan with cooking spray and spread mixture in pan; bake for 15 minutes.

4.  While crust bakes heat a skillet and season beef with basil, salt, pepper, cumin, Italian seasoning, and turmeric; cook for 10 minutes.

5.  Remove crust from oven and cool for 10 minutes. Top crust with tomato sauce and cheese along with the meat.

6.  Bake for an additional 10 minutes and broil for 5 minutes.

7.  Cool, slice and serve.

*[Calories 145 | Total Fats 11.3g | Net Carbs: 1.2g | Protein 8.2g]*

## No-Bun Hamburger

[Total Time: 20 MIN| Serve: 2]

*Ingredients:*

*½ lb. ground beef*

*½ onion, chopped*

*1 tspvsalt*

*1 tsp pepper*

*4 slices American cheddar*

*4 bacon strips, cooked and chopped*

*4 pcs butter or romaine lettuce leaves*

*4 tbsp mayonnaise*

Directions:

1. Heat a cast iron skillet over medium heat. Add the ground beef and sauté with the onions. Cook until the beef is no longer pink.

2. Season the beef with the garlic powder, salt, and pepper.

3. Reduce the heat to low and then top the beef with the slices of cheese. Cover and cook for 3 minutes, or until the cheese has melted

4. Scoop the cooked "burger patties" on the top of the lettuce leaves and dollop mayonnaise on top.

5. Serve immediately.

   *[Calories 224 | Total Fats 7.1g | Net Carbs: 3.2g | Protein 34.8g | Fiber 0.9g]*

## Keto Ham and Cheese Stromboli

[Total Time: 35 MIN| Serve: 4]

*Ingredients:*

*1 ¼ cups mozzarella cheese*

*3 tbsp coconut flour*

*1 tsp Italian seasoning*

*3 ½ oz cheddar cheese*

*4 tbsp almond flour*

*1 egg*

*4 oz ham*

*Salt*

*Black pepper*

Directions:

1.  Preheat oven to 400⁰F. Place mozzarella into a microwave safe dish and melt for 1 minute, stirring occasionally.

2.  Mix flour and seasoning together in a bowl then add melted cheese and combine thoroughly.

3.  Cool for a minute then add egg and mix together. Place parchment paper on a baking sheet and place mozzarella dough onto paper, top with another paper and use a rolling pin to flatten.

4.  Use a knife to slice dough diagonally from edge to middle of the dough, leaving 4 inches of dough unsliced.

5.  Place ham and cheese on unsliced section of dough and cover with sliced section

6.  Bake for 15-20 minutes until the top is browned. Serve warm.

    *[Calories 306 | Total Fats 21.8g | Net Carbs: 4.7g | Protein 25.6g | Fiber: 3.8g]*

## *Spaghetti Squash Lasagna Dish*

[Total Time: 1 HR 30 MIN| Serve: 14]

*Ingredients:*

*2 ¹ᐟ² lbs. ground beef*

*2 large Spaghetti Squash*

*7 ounces whole milk Ricotta Cheese*

*7 ounces Mozzarella cheese, sliced*

*4 cups Marinara sauce*

*Coconut or olive oil for greasing*

Directions:

1. Preheat oven to 375°F. Grease a large baking dish with coconut or olive oil.

2. Split the Spaghetti Squash and lay face down into a large glass dish and fill with water. Bake for 40-45 minutes.

3. While the Spaghetti Squash is cooking, in a large saucepan cook the ground meat and the marinara sauce. Once combined, set aside.

4. When the Spaghetti Squash is done scrape the meat of the squash to from spaghetti.

5. Assemble the lasagna in a large greased pan, start with a layer of Spaghetti Squash, then the meat sauce, then slices of mozzarella, then ricotta, then repeats until ingredients are exhausted.

6.   Bake for 30-35 minutes until the top layer of cheese is browning. Serve hot or keep refrigerated.

*[Calories 437 | Total Fats 27.7g | Net Carbs: 16.4g | Protein 28g | Fiber: 1.9g]*

## *Italian Sausage and Spinach Casserole*
[Total Time: 1 HR 5 MIN| Serve: 10]

*Ingredients:*

*16 oz. spicy Italian sausage*

*2 ½ cups frozen spinach*

*12 eggs*

*8 oz. Cheddar*

*1 onion*

*9 oz. Cherry Tomatoes*

*1 green pepper, chopped*

*12 Tbsp Heavy Cream*

*Garlic powder*

*Onion Powder*

*Salt and ground pepper to taste*

*Coconut or olive oil*

Directions:

1.   Preheat oven to 350⁰F. Grease casserole dish with coconut or olive oil.

2.  In microwave cook the spinach. Chop the spicy Italian sausage and cook in a frying pan until browned. Remove to the big bowl and set aside.

3.  In the same frying pan, cook the sliced onion and pepper. Transfer to the bowl with spinach.

4.  Whisk together the eggs, spices and a heavy cream. Add the cheese to the bowl and combine, then add the egg mixture and combine.

5.  Transfer to a greased casserole dish and add cherry tomatoes.

6.  Cook in preheated oven for 50 minutes. Serve hot.

    *[Calories 343 | Total Fats 25g | Net Carbs: 6.2g | Protein 22g | Fiber: 2.5g]*

## Sausage & Cheese Bombs

[Total Time: 25 MIN| Serve: 12]

*Ingredients:*

*12. oz. pork sausage*

*¾ cup sharp cheddar cheese, shredded*

*12 mozzarella cheese cubes*

Directions:

1.  Crumble the sausage and combine with the shredded cheese in a bowl.

2.  Divide into 12 patties and place 1 mozzarella cube at the center of each patty.

3.   Cover the cheese with the meat and create a ball.

4.   Heat your fryer up to 375 and fry the meatballs until golden brown.

5.   Serve with a keto-friendly marinara sauce on the side.

*[Calories 173 | Total Fats 14g | Net Carbs: 1g | Protein 10g]*


## *Mediterranean Pecorino Romano Breaded Cutlets*
[Total Time: 30 MIN| Serve: 3]

*Ingredients:*

*6 pork cutlets*

*½ cup grated Pecorino Romano cheese*

*2 Tbsp fresh lemon juice*

*2 Tbsp water*

*1 Tbsp olive oil*

*1 Tbsp green pepper, minced*

*1 Tbsp garlic, minced*

*Salt and ground black pepper to taste*

Directions:

1.   Heat a greasing frying pan to medium.

2.   In a bowl pour water, lemon juice, olive oil, minced pepper, and garlic. Season the salt and pepper to taste. Mix well.

3.   In a separate bowl pour grated Pecorino Romano cheese.

4. Dip each cutlet first in liquid dressing and then in cheese.

5. Cook cutlets in pan for about 15-20 minutes. Serve hot.

   *[Calories 395 | Total Fats 38g | Net Carbs: 2.5g | Protein 9.1g | Fiber 0.16g]*

## Slow-Cook Pumpkin Chili

[Total Time: 1 Hr 20 MIN| Serve: 8]

*Ingredients:*

*2 lbs. ground beef*

*1 can (15 oz.) pumpkin puree*

*1 Tbsp pumpkin pie spice*

*3 cups 100% tomato juice*

*3 tomatoes, diced*

*1 red bell pepper*

*1 yellow onion*

*2 tsp cumin*

*1 Tbsp chili powder*

*2 tsp cayenne pepper*

*Ghee or coconut oil*

Directions:

1. In a large frying pan greased with ghee or coconut oil, brown the meat over medium heat.

2.  Chop the onion and pepper and add into the pot with the meat. Cook 3-5 minutes or until the onions become translucent.

3.  Add in the rest of the ingredients and let simmer on LOW for 30 minutes.

4.  Season chili with salt and pepper to taste and cook for another 30 minutes.

5.  Serve hot.

    *[Calories 354 | Total Fats 25g | Net Carbs: 9.8g | Protein 21g | Fiber: 2.14 g]*

## Monterey Jack Steak

[Total Time: 20 MIN| Serve: 4]

*Ingredients:*

*1 lb. shaved steak*

*4 slices Monterey Jack cheese*

*2 Tbsp mayonnaise*

*1 Tbsp Dijon mustard*

*¼ cup chopped green peppers*

*¼ up chopped onions*

*1 Tbsp minced garlic*

*1 Tbsp olive oil*

*1 Tbsp ghee*

Directions:

1. In a large frying pan add ghee and olive oil to warm over medium heat. Add onions, green peppers, and garlic. Cook until soft, about 2-3 minutes. Add shaved steak and cook until browned several minutes.

2. Turn heat down to low. Add Dijon mustard and mayonnaise and mix.

3. Add Monterey Jack cheese on top of the steak and let melt until cheese is melted throughout about 1 minute.

4. Serve hot.

   *[Calories 345 | Total Fats 25g | Net Carbs: 4.3g | Protein 24g | Fiber 0.4g]*

## *Low-Carb Cheesy Pizza*

[Total Time: 20 MIN| Serve: 7]

*Ingredients:*

*1 lb. ground beef*

*2 beef sausage*

*1 cup chopped Romaine lettuce*

*2 Tbsp yellow onions*

*3 Tbsp chopped dill pickle*

*1 ½ cups Parmesan cheese*

*½ cup Colby cheese, shredded*

1 ½ cups Cheddar, shredded

¼ Tbsp paprika

¼ tsp Old Bay seasoning

¼ tsp garlic powder

¼ tsp onion powder

2 Tbsp organic Thousand Island dressing

Mustard to taste

¼ tsp sea salt

¼ tsp ground black pepper

Olive oil

2 Tbsp water

Directions:

1.  In a frying pan greased with olive oil, add 1 cup Parmesan cheese evenly and then on top, 1 cup shredded Cheddar.

2.  Leave to cook 2-3 minutes; use a spatula to lift the edges and underneath of the pizza, and slide out onto a flat surface. Allow cooling.

3.  Repeat the same process, for the second pizza crust.

4.  Once done, set both cheese crusts aside.

5.  Use a spatula and evenly spread Thousand Island dressing over the cheese crusts

6.  In a frying pan add ground beef and cook until browned. Add old bay seasoning, garlic powder,

onion powder paprika, 2 tbsp water,  salt, ground black pepper to taste. Mixoand set to simmer on low.

7.  Finally, add in chopped hot dogs into slices and simmer for about 4-5 minutes.

8.  Place chopped lettuce over your pizza crust.

9.  In a bowl, place your pickles, onions, Colby cheese, and set aside.

10. On top of each cheese crust, add about a cup of the ground meat and hot dog mixture and spread evenly. Sprinkle with onions and pickles.

11. Drizzle mustard on top.

12. Sprinkle with more cheese if you like and serve.

*[Calories 511 | Total Fats 39g | Net Carbs: 2.7g | Protein 33g | Fiber 0.4g]*

## *Spicy Spinach Casserole*
[Total Time: 60 MIN| Serve: 10]

*Ingredients:*

*2 ½ cups spinach, drained*

*2 lbs. ground pork/beef*

*16 oz. cream cheese*

*10 Tbsp sour cream*

*8 oz. Emmenthal Cheese, shredded*

*2 cups pepper sauce*

*1 onion*

*1 red pepper*

*4 tsp taco seasoning*

*Sliced jalapeños to taste*

Directions:

1. Preheat oven to 350⁰F. Grease one 8" square and a 9x13 baking dish.

2. Chop and sauté some jalapenos with chopped peppers and onions. Transfer to a bowl and set aside.

3. Add the spinach to the pan and cook until thawed completely. Move the spinach to the prep bowl

4. In a frying pan, add ground pork/meat and cook until browned well. Add taco seasoning and mix. oRemove from fire and setoaside.

5. In a bowl, add sour cream, mozzarella, and cream cheese. Add in peppers, onion, spinach and ground meat.

6. Transfer this mix to prepared and greased baking dish and bake for 40 minutes.

7. Serve hot or cold.

   *[Calories 460 | Total Fats 37g | Net Carbs: 5.3g | Protein 25g | Fiber 0.8g]*

## Bolognese Stuffed Spaghetti Squash

[Total Time: 1 HR 40 MIN| Serve: 5]

*Ingredients:*

*1 lb. ground beef*

*2 ½ cups Spaghetti squash*

*1 egg*

*3/4 cup Marinara Sauce*

*1 cup grated Parmesan cheese*

*1 cups shredded mozzarella cheese*

*1 tsp chili powder*

*½ tsp oregano*

*½ tsp parsley (fresh and chopped)*

*½ tsp basil*

*1 tsp crushed red pepper flakes*

*2 tsp of garlic minced*

*Sea salt and ground fresh pepper to taste*

*Ghee*

Directions:

1.  Preheat oven to 350⁰F.

2.  Roast your spaghetti squash in the oven for about one hour.

3.  In a saucepan, heat Marinara sauce; add oregano, parsley, basil and red pepper flakes. Cover and let simmer for a few minutes. Mix meatball ingredients in a bowl and roll into quarter-sized mini meatballs.

4. In a frying pan heat, the ghee and cook meatballs covered. After 3 minutes, flip when halfway browned.

5. Once the meatballs are cooked through, transfer them into the sauce.

6. In a small bread pan, layer spaghetti squash, sauce, meatballs and mozzarella.

7. Bake on 25 for 30 minutes. Serve hot.

*[Calories 446 | Total Fats 30g | Net Carbs: 9.1g| Protein 32g | Fiber0.9g]*

## Tender Sweet 'n' Sour Pork Chops

[Total Time: 1 HR 10 MIN| Serve: 10]

*Ingredients:*

*4.4 lbs. pork chops*

*1 cup Apple cider vinegar*

*1 cup Erythritol*

*4 Tbsp Soy Sauce*

*1 cup Apple Cider Vinegar*

*1 tsp ginger*

*1 tsp pepper*

*Coconut or olive oil for greasing*

Directions:

1. Preheat oven to 350°F.

2. In a food processor, add all of the ingredients (except the pork chops).

3. Blend well to make the marinade.

4. In a greased pan place all of the pork chops and pour the marinade over it.

5. Cook for 60 minutes in a preheated oven flipping after 30 minutes.

6. Once ready place chops on a serving plate and enjoys your lunch.

*[Calories 307 | Total Fats 6g | Net Carbs: 11.43g | Protein 45g | Fiber 0.08g]*

## Low Carb Cheesy Pizza

[Total Time: 55 MIN| Serve: 12]

*Ingredients:*

*½ lb ground beef*

*2 eggs*

*1 tsp garlic powder*

*¼ tsp basil*

*¼ tsp turmeric*

*8 oz cream cheese*

*1 Chorizo sausage*

*¼ cup parmesan cheese, grated*

*½ tsp cumin*

*½ tsp Italian seasoning*

¾ *cup tomato sauce*

*Salt*

*Black pepper*

Directions:

1. Set oven to 375⁰F.

2. Put cream cheese, eggs, garlic powder, parmesan cheese and black pepper in a bowl and use a mixer to blend until smooth.

3. Grease a baking pan and pour in cheese mixture and spread evenly; bake for 15 minutes.

4. Put beef into a skillet and cook for 5 minutes then add Italian seasoning, basil, salt, black pepper, cumin, and turmeric. Cook for 10 minutes or until thoroughly cooked.

5. Take crust from oven and cool for 10 minutes then top with tomato sauce and cheese. Return to oven and bake for 10 minutes until cheese melts then top with beef.

6. Broil for an additional 5 minutes. Take from oven and cool for 10 minutes.

7. Slice and serve.

*[Calories 145 | Total Fats 11.3g | Net Carbs: 1.2g | Protein 8.2g | Fiber 3g]*

## Grilled Ham and Cheese Sandwich

[Total Time: 30 MIN| Serve: 2]

*Ingredients:*

*For buns:*

*2 eggs*

*1 ½ tbsp butter, salted*

*1 tsp coconut flour*

*¾ cup almond flour*

*2 tbsp coconut oil*

*1 tsp baking powder*

*¼ tsp salt*

*Filling:*

*4 Deli Ham slices*

*2 cheddar cheese, slices*

*1 tbsp butter, salted*

*2 Muenster cheese, slices*

Directions:

1. Set oven to 350$^0$F.

2. Place almond flour, baking powder in a bowl and mix together.

3. Put coconut oil and butter in a microwavable dish and heat until melted then add to dry mix. Combine until mixture gets doughy.

4.  Beat eggs and add to dough mixture then put in coconut flour.

5.  Grease cupcake molds and add batter to each about ¾ ways filled. Baked for 18 minutes and take from oven, allow to cool and slice into two horizontally.

6.  Use cheese and ham to fill buns, melt butter in a skillet and place sandwiches in the pan. Cook for 3 minutes on each side until golden and cheese melts.

7.  Serve.

    *[Calories 272 | Total Fats 24.2g | Net Carbs: 1.8g | Protein 11.3g | Fiber 3.8g]*


## Polish Sausage, Bacon & Broccoli Casserole
[Total Time: 45 MIN| Serve: 8]

*Ingredients:*

*1.1 lbs beef sausage*

*½ head of broccoli*

*8 slices of bacon*

*½ cups cream*

*1 tbsp Dijon mustard*

*1 cup cheddar cheese, grated*

Directions:

1.  Preheat oven to 350⁰F.

2.  Slice the sausage and place in a small baking dish.

3.  Slice the bacon and add to the sausage.

4.  Break the broccoli into florets and arrange between the meat.

5.  Mix the cream and mustard in a bowl and pour it all over the casserole, then top with the cheese.

6.  Bake in the oven for 35 minutes.

*[Calories 300 | Total Fats 25g | Net Carbs: 3g | Protein 20g]*

## Cheesy Bacon Spinach Dip

[Total Time: 1 HR 15 MIN| Serve: 5]

*Ingredients:*

*2 ½ cups cheddar cheese, shredded*

*2 tbsp chipotle seasoning*

*30 bacon slices*

*2 tsp Mrs. Dash seasoning*

*5 cups spinach*

Directions:

1.  Set oven to 375⁰F.

2.  Place bacon in a weaving pattern on a baking sheet lined with foil and season with spices.

3.  Top bacon with cheese leaving a 1-inch space all around the edge. Add spinach and push it down and roll the bacon together into a log.

4.  Sprinkle with salt and place into oven for 60 minutes.

5. Cool for 15 minutes and slice.

6. Serve.

   *[Calories 432 | Total Fats 38.2g | Net Carbs: 3g | Protein 32.8g | Fiber 3g]*

## Savoury Mince

[Total Time: 20 MIN| Serve: 5]

*Ingredients:*

*4 tbsp coconut oil*

*2.2 lbs Beef/Chicken/Lamb/Pork/Ostrich mince*

*2 onions finely diced*

*4 cups vegetables (green/red/yellow/orange peppers, mushroom, tomatoes, celery, baby marrows, and spinach) finely diced*

*4 carrots finely grated*

*1 packet gluten-free gravy*

*½ cup tomato paste*

*1 cup chicken stock*

Directions:

1. Heat coconut oil in a pan and fry chopped onion, Add beef mince with and tomato paste and fry.

2. Add chopped vegetables and grated carrot to the cooked mince.

3. Continue to cook on a low heat until the vegetables are well cooked.

4. If your mixture seems to be drying out, keep adding chicken stock to keep at the right consistency.

5. The longer you cook this mixture, the more the flavors will infuse through the mince.

6. Add gluten-free gravy.

   *[Calories 596 | Total Fats 14.3g | Net Carbs: 28g | Protein 65.5g | Fiber: 10.7g]*

## Chorizo-Stuffed Bell Peppers

[Total Time: 45 MIN| Serve: 2]

*Ingredients:*

*3 large bell peppers, cut in half, core and seeds removed*

*½ lb. spicy chorizo sausage, crumbled*

*2 cloves of garlic*

*1 onion, chopped*

*6 organic eggs*

*¼ cup almond milk, unsweetened*

*1 cup cheddar cheese, shredded*

*½ tbsp ghee*

*Salt and pepper to taste*

Directions:

1. Set oven to 350⁰F.

2. Heat the ghee in a non-stick pan over medium heat and cook the chorizo crumbles. Set aside.

3. Using the same pan, add the onions and garlic and sauté for a few minutes. Turn off the heat and set aside.

4. In a bowl, stir together the eggs, milk, cheddar, and season with salt and pepper.

5. Add the chorizo into the bowl with the eggs and stir well.

6. Place the bell pepper halves in an oven-safe dish filled with a ¼ inch of water.

7. Scoop the chorizo and egg mixture into the bell peppers and place the dish into the oven to bake for 35 minutes.

8. Serve warm.

*[Calories 631 | Total Fats 46g | Net Carbs: 13g | Protein 44g | Fiber 3.5g]*


## Kalamata Olives & Sour Sausages with Shallots
[Total Time: 30 MIN| Serve: 6]

*Ingredients:*

*1 lb sausages chopped*

*4 shallots, finely chopped*

*½ cup lemon juice (2 lemons)*

*16 black and green Kalamata olives*

*2 Tbsp whole grain mustard*

*4 Tbsp extra virgin olive oil*

*Saltvand ground black pepper to taste*

Directions:

1. Preheat oven to 400°F. Grease a roasting pan and place in the sausages and chopped shallots.

2. Roast for 20 minutes.

3. When ready, remove the meat from the sausages and season with salt and freshly ground pepper to taste.

4. Pour the lemon juice into the roasting tin.

5. Add the mustard and chopped olives and simmer gently for 2-3 minutes. Pour lemon mixture over the sausages and shallots.

6. Place on serving plate and serve.

   *[Calories 408 | Total Fats 16.67g | Net Carbs: 6.78g | Protein 18.48g | Fiber: 0.42g]*


## *Persian Sour 'n' Spicy Goat Kebab*
[Total Time: 25 MIN| Serve: 2]

*Ingredients:*

*1 lb boneless goat loin, cut into cubes*

*2 Tbsp lime juice (freshly squeezed)*

*1 cup coconut yogurt*

*¼ tsp ground ginger*

*3/4 tsp turmeric*

*½ tsp ground cumin*

1 Tbsp ground coriander

½ tsp salt

Skewers

Directions:

1. In a medium bowl, stir together coconut yogurt, lime juice, and all seasonings; mix well.

2. Add the goat meat cubes to the bowl, stir to coat with the marinade, cover and refrigerate for 6-8 hours.

3. Remove the meat from the marinade, pat lightly with paper towels to dry.

4. Place meat evenly on the skewers. Grill over medium-hot coals, turning frequently, for about 10 minutes until nicely brown.

5. Serve and enjoy.

   *[Calories 342.93 | Total Fats 9.79g | Net Carbs: 7.96g | Protein 26.77g | Fiber: 1.25g]*

## Meaty Italian Bagels

[Total Time: 60 MIN| Serve: 2]

*Ingredients:*

*3 small onions, minced*

*2 tbsp organic butter*

*4 lbs ground pork*

*4 organic eggs*

1 ¼ cups all-natural tomato sauce

2 tsp paprika

Salt and pepper to taste

Directions:

1. Set the oven at 400°F.

2. Melt the butter in a non-stick pan over medium heat. Add the minced onions and sauté for a few minutes until the onions turn translucent. Set aside

3. In a large bowl, combine the ground pork, eggs, and tomato sauce. Season with salt, pepper, paprika and then add the sautéed onions.

4. Combine the ingredients using your hands and then form into 12 balls.

5. Flatten the middle of the ball to make it look like a bagel and then place on top of a baking sheet lined with parchment paper.

6. Bake in the oven to bake for 40 minutes or until cooked through.

   [Calories 805 | Total Fats 26.4g | Net Carbs: 9.9g | Protein 126g | Fiber: 2.7 g]


## Mutton Madras

[Total Time: 5 HR 20 MIN| Serve: 8]

Ingredients:

8 Fatty lamb chops

6 tbsp Coconut Milk

2 cups water

3 tbsp Red Curry Paste

2 tbsp Thai fish sauce

1 tbsp dried onion flakes

2 tbsp dried Thai or fresh red chilies

1 tbsp Xylitol

1 tbsp ground cumin

1 tbsp ground coriander

1/8 tsp ground cloves

1/8 tsp ground nutmeg

1 tbsp ground ginger

To Serve:

2 tbsp coconut milk powder

1 tbsp red curry paste

2 tbsp Xylitol

¼ cup cashews, roughly chopped

¼ cup fresh cilantro, chopped

## Directions:

1.  Place the raw lamb chops in a large slow cooker.

2.  Add the 6 tbsp coconut milk, water, 3 tbsp red curry paste, fish sauce, onion flakes, chilies, 1 tbsp Xylitol, ginger, nutmeg, cloves, coriander, and cumin. Cover with lid and cook on high for 5 hours.

3. Just before serving, remove the meat from slow cooker and place on another dish. Then stir into the sauce the 2 tbsp coconut milk powder, 1 tbsp curry paste, 2 tbsp sweetener, and 1/4 tsp xanthan gum (if using).

4. Shred the meat and stir into the sauce, along with cashews. Garnish with coriander before serving.

*[Calories 190 | Total Fats 11g | Net Carbs: 4g | Protein 18g]*

## Spinach 'n' Lamb Curry

[Total Time: 8 HR 25 MIN| Serve: 8]

*Ingredients:*

*1/3 cup coconut or olive oil*

*3 yellow onions, chopped*

*4 cloves garlic, peeled and minced*

*2cm piece of ginger, peeled and grated*

*2 tsp ground cumin*

*1 ½ tsp cayenne pepper*

*1 ½ tsp ground turmeric*

*2 cups beefvstock, preferably high quality*

*3.3 lbs leg of lamb, cut into 2cm cubes*

*Salt*

*6 cups baby spinach*

*2 cups plain full-fat yogurt*

Directions:

1. In a large frying pan over medium-high heat, warm oil. Add onions and garlic, and sauté until golden, about 5 minutes. Stir in ginger, cumin, cayenne, and turmeric and sauté until fragrant, or for about 30 seconds.

2. Pour in broth scraping up the browned bits on the bottom. When broth comes to a boil, remove the pan from heat.

3. Put lamb in a slow cooker, and sprinkle with 1 tbsp. salt. Add contents of frying pan. Cover and cook on high-heat setting for 4 hours or low-heat setting for 8 hours.

4. Add baby spinach to pot and cook, stirring occasionally, until spinach is wilted, about 5 minutes. Just before serving, stir in 1 1/3 cups yogurt. Season to taste with salt.

*[Calories 304 | Total Fats 16g | Net Carbs: 5g | Protein 32g]*

## *Balsamic Roast Pork*
[Total Time: 8 HR 15 MIN| Serve: 4]

*Ingredients:*

*1 lb. pork roast*

*½ cup balsamic vinegar*

*1/3 cup honey*

*2 tsp fresh rosemary*

*½ tsp thyme (Dried)*

*2 bay leaves*

*2 tsp salt*

*¼ tsp black pepper*

Directions:

1. Place pork roast in the slow cooker.

2. Mix all ingredients in a bowl and pour over roast.

3. Cook on low for 6-8 hours, or high for 4-6, depending on the size of the roast.

4. Remove the cooked roast from the slow-cooker.

5. Cover and keep warm.

6. Pour the remaining sauce from slow cooker into a saucepan and bring to a boil.

7. Let it reduce by about half.

8. Slice the roast and pour the sauce over top.

   *[Calories 379 | Total Fats 11.45g | Net Carbs: 32.7g | Protein 35g]*

## *Bolognese Mince*

[Total Time: 6 HR 20 MIN| Serve: 8]

*Ingredients:*

*2.2 lbs beef mince*

*2 brown onions, diced*

*4 cloves garlic, crushed*

*1 cup tomato paste*

*2 tbsp chicken stock powder or 2 Knorr Jelly Pots*

*1 tin tomatovsoup*

*1 tin diced tomato*

*¼ cup sweet chili sauce*

*1 tbsp oregano*

*2 bay leaves*

*2 cups water*

*1 cup finely grated carrot*

*3-4 finely chopped sticks of celery*

*2 cups finely chopped mushrooms*

Directions:

1.  In a frying pan, add the olive oil and heat. Brown the beef and add the onions and garlic. Cook for 2 minutes more.

2.  Mix the tomato paste into the pan and cook for another 2 minutes.

3.  Pour all of the mixtures into the slow cooker and add the rest of the ingredients and stir.

4.  Cook on low for 6 hours or high for 3 hours.

    *[Calories 187 | Total Fats 5.2g | Net Carbs: 8g | Protein 27g]*

## Smoked Pork Cassoulet

[Total Time: 5 HR 15 MIN| Serve: 6]

*Ingredients:*

*1 pack bacon, fried and then crumbled*

*2 cups chopped onion*

*1 tsp dried thyme*

*½ tsp dried rosemary*

*3 garlic cloves, crushed*

*½ tsp salt*

*½ tsp freshly ground black pepper*

*2 cans diced tomatoes, drained*

*1.1 lbs boneless pork loin roast, trimmed and cut into 2cm cubes*

*1.2 lbs smoked sausage, cut into 1cm cubes*

*8 tsp finely shredded fresh Parmesan cheese*

*8 tsp chopped fresh flat-leaf parsley*

Directions:

1. Fry bacon onion, thyme, rosemary, and garlic, then add salt, pepper, and tomatoes; bring to a boil.

2. Remove from heat.

3. Place all ingredients in the slow cooker, alternating the meat with the tomato sauce until finished. Cover and cook on low for 5 hours. Sprinkle with Parmesan cheese and parsley when cooked

*[Calories 258 | Total Fats 12.6g | Net Carbs: 10.8g | Protein 27g]*

## Tomato Bredie

[Total Time: 4 HR 20 MIN| Serve: 8]

*Ingredients:*

*1 tbsp olive oil*

*3.3 lbs or mutton chops or 1.5kgs of stewing lamb*

*2 tbsp almondvflour, psyllium husk or finely ground chia seeds*

*1 large onion,vchopped*

*3.3 lbs fresh tomatoes, finely chopped*

*1 tsp salt*

*1/2 tsp freshly ground black pepper*

*2 bay leaves*

*1 tsp Xylitol*

*1 tbsp white vinegar*

*1 dash Worcestershire sauce*

*1 cube beef or lamb stock*

Directions:

1.  Heat oil over medium-high heat in a large, heavy-bottomed saucepan.

2.  Dredge meat in almond flour and cook in hot oil until well browned.

3.  Stir in onions, and cook for about 5 minutes or until soft. Mix in tomatoes.

4.  Season with salt, black pepper, white peppercorns, bay leaves, xylitol, vinegar, Worcestershire sauce, and beef bouillon cube.

5.  Cover, reduce heat and simmer for 3-4 hours on low.

    *[Calories 385 | Total Fats 15g | Net Carbs: 9g | Protein 50g]*

## Soups & Stews

### Hearty Lemon Chicken Stew
[Total Time: 6 HR 30 MIN| Serve: 10]

*Ingredients:*

*2 carrots, chopped*

*2 ribs celery, chopped*

*1 onion, chopped*

*20 large green olives*

*4 cloves garlic, crushed*

*2 bay leaves*

*½ tsp dried oregano*

*¼ tsp salt*

*¼ tsp pepper*

*12 boneless skinless chicken thighs*

*¾ cup chicken stock*

*¼ cup almond flour or psyllium husk or finely ground*

*Chia seeds*

*2 tbsp lemon juice*

*½ cup chopped fresh parsley*

*Grated zest of 1 lemon*

Directions:

1.  In slow cooker, combine carrots, celery, onion, olives, garlic, bay leaves, oregano, salt, and pepper.

2.  Arrange chicken pieces on top of vegetables. Add broth and ¾ cup water. Cover and cook on low for 5-1/2 to 6 hours or until juices run clear when chicken is pierced. Discard bay leaves.

3.  Whisk flour with 1 cup of the cooking liquid until smooth; whisk in lemon juice. Pour mixture into slow cooker; cook, covered, on high until thickened, about 15 minutes.

4.  Mix parsley with lemon zest; serve sprinkled over chicken mixture. Enjoy!

    *[Calories 331 | Total Fats 15.7g | Net Carbs: 3.9g | Protein 40.5g | Fiber 1.2g]*

## Beef Chuck Cabbage Stew

[Total Time: 9 HR 15 MIN| Serve: 6]

*Ingredients:*

*1 packet frozen baby carrots*

*2 medium onions, roughly chopped*

*1 small cabbage cored, and cut into 8 wedges*

*8 garlic cloves, peeled and smashed*

*2 bay leaves*

*8 pieces of beef chuck with marrow*

*Salt and freshly ground pepper to taste*

*2 tins diced tomatoes, drained*

*1 cup chicken stock*

Directions:

1.   Place the baby carrots and chopped onions into the bottom of the slow cooker.

2.   Layer the cabbage wedges on top.

3.   Add crushed garlic cloves and bay leaves

4.   Season the beef shanks with salt and pepper (by the way, feel free to be pretty heavy-handed with the S&P).

5.   Add beef shanks on top of vegetables.

6.   Pour in the diced tomatoes and broth before putting on the lid.

7.   Set the slow cooker on low for 9 hours.

   *[Calories 234 | Total Fats 16g | Net Carbs: 5g | Protein 16g]*

## *Hearty Beef Stew*

[Total Time: 8 HR 20 MIN| Serve: 6]

*Ingredients:*

*2.2 lbs stewing beef*

*3 Tbsp olive oil*

*2 cups beef stock*

*1 packet streaky bacon – cooked crisp and crumbled*

*2 cans diced tomatoes – juice drained*

*2 cups mixed bell peppers – chopped*

*2 cups mushrooms – quartered*

*2 ribs celery – chopped*

*1 large carrot – chopped*

*1 small onion – chopped*

*4 large cloves garlic – minced*

*2 Tbsp organic tomato paste*

*2 Tbsp Worcestershire sauce*

*2 tsp sea salt*

*1 ½ tsp black pepper*

*1 tsp garlic powder*

*1 tsp onion powder*

*1 tsp dried oregano*

Directions:

1. Set slow cooker on low.

2. In a large pan over medium heat, sear the beef in olive oil, browning on both sides. Transfer to slow cooker.

3. Pour beef stock, bacon, tomatoes, bell peppers, mushrooms, celery, carrot, onion, garlic, tomato paste, Worcestershire sauce, sea salt, black pepper, garlic powder, onion powder, and dried oregano into the slow cooker.

4. Cover and cook on low 6-8 hours.

   *[Calories 280 | Total Fats 6g | Net Carbs: 20g | Protein 18g]*

## Curried Chicken Stew

[Total Time: 8 HR 20 MIN| Serve: 8]

*Ingredients:*

*8 bone-in chicken thighs*

*2 tbsp olive oil or coconut oil*

*6 carrots cut into 2-inch pieces*

*1 sweet onion cut into thin wedges*

*1 cup unsweetened coconut milk*

*¼ cup milk (or hot) curry paste*

*Toasted almonds, coriander, and fresh green or red chili*

## Directions:

1. Cook chicken in a pan skin side down, in hot olive oil for 8 minutes, or until browned.

2. Remove from heat; drain and discard fat.

3. In a slow cooker combine carrots and onion.

4. Whisk together half the coconut milk and the curry paste; pour over carrots and onion

5. Place chicken, skin side up on top of vegetables, pour over olive oil from pan.

6. Cover and cook on high for 3.5 to 4 hours or on low for 7 to 8 hours.

7. Remove chicken from slow cooker. Skim excess fat from sauce in the cooker, and then stir in remaining coconut milk.

8.  Serve stew in bowls. Top each serving with toasted almonds, coriander, fresh chili and a dollop of yogurt or crème Fraiche.

    *[Calories 321 | Total Fats 22g | Net Carbs: 20g | Protein 14g]*

## Curried Cauliflower & Chicken Stew
[Total Time: 6 HR 20 MIN| Serve: 8]

*Ingredients:*

*3½ tbsp coconut oil*

*1 bunch fresh mint or coriander leaves, chopped*

*1 head cauliflower, broken into large florets*

*Freshly ground black pepper*

*1½ tbsp salt*

*6 bone-in skinless chicken thighs, about 1.1kg*

*2 cups whole milk plain yogurt*

*3 cups chicken stock, low-sodium canned*

*½ cup prepared red curry paste (depending on heat required)*

*5-cm piece fresh ginger, minced*

*6 cloves garlic, minced*

*1 lemon cut in wedges*

Directions:

1.  Heat the oil; add the garlic and ginger and cook. Add the curry paste and continue to cook. Whisk the broth in the pan; then pour the liquid into a slow cooker. Whisk the yogurt into the liquid.

2. Season the chicken all over with salt and pepper.

3. Add the chicken and remaining salt to the slow cooker. Cover and cook on high for 6 hours, adding cauliflower about halfway through cooking.

4. Scatter freshly torn mint or coriander on top. Serve with a wedge of lemon.

*[Calories 343 | Total Fats 15g | Net Carbs: 31g | Protein 23g]*

## Farmhouse Lamb & Cabbage Stew
[Total Time: 6 HR 50 MIN| Serve: 8]

*Ingredients:*

*2 tbsp olive oil or coconut oil*

*1.1 lb lamb chops, bone in*

*1 lamb or beef stock cube*

*2 cups water*

*1 cabbage, finely chopped*

*1 onion, sliced*

*2 carrots, chopped*

*2 sticks celery, chopped*

*1 tsp dried thyme*

*1 tbsp balsamic vinegar*

*1 tbsp almond flour or psyllium husk*

Directions:

1. Set the slow cooker to low.

2. Heat oil in a large frying pan and brown the lamb chops.

3. Add lamb to the slow cooker with remaining ingredients, mix until ingredients are evenly distributed.

4. Cook on low for 6- to hours. Then remove bones from lamb.

5. For thicker a sauce, 30 minutes before serving ladle ¼ cup of the sauce into a small bowl and whisk almond flour into it with a fork. Return mixture to the slow cooker bowl, stir through and leave for a further 30minutes.

*[Calories 180 | Total Fats 4g | Net Carbs: 9g | Protein 26g]*

## Seafood Stew

[Total Time: 6 HR 50 MIN| Serve: 8]

*Ingredients:*

*1 tbsp olive oil*

*2 onions, diced*

*4 stalks celery, chopped*

*4 garlic cloves, minced*

*1 tsp dried oregano*

*½ tsp ground black pepper*

*1 tbsp tomato paste*

*1 tbsp flour*

*3 cups chicken stock*

*1 can tomato, onion and chili mix*

*1 -2 cup tomato cocktail juice*

*4 chicken breasts cut into bite-size pieces*

*2 packets mixed frozen seafood; you can add extra mussels in at the end*

*2 peppers (red and green)*

*1 jalapeno pepper, chopped*

*¼ cup parsley, chopped*

*1 tsp chili powder*

*1 pinch cayenne pepper*

*1 tbsp butter*

Directions:

1. In a large pan heat the olive oil and fry onions and celery

2. Add garlic, oregano, peppercorns.

3. Stir in tomato paste and almond flour and cook another minute.

4. Add chicken stock, tomatoes and tomato juice and bring to a boil. Continue to cook for about 3-5 more minutes. Remove from heat and transfer mixture to slow cooker.

5. Add chicken and stir to combine. Cover and cook on high for 3 hours or low for 6 hours.

6. Stir in mixed bags of frozen and parsley. Cover and cook on high for 30 minutes

*[Calories 177 | Total Fats 4g | Net Carbs: 15g | Protein 21g]*

## Rosemary Garlic Beef Stew

[Total Time: 4 HR 20 MIN| Serve: 8]

*Ingredients:*

*4 medium carrots, sliced*

*4 sticks celery, sliced*

*1 medium onion, diced*

*2 tbsp olive oil*

*4 garlic cloves, minced*

*1.5 lbs beef stewing meat (shin or chuck)*

*Salt and pepper*

*¼ cup almond flour*

*2 cups beef stock*

*2 tbsp Dijon mustard*

*1 tbsp Worcestershire sauce*

*1 tbsp soy sauce*

*1 tbsp xylitol*

*½ tbsp dried rosemary*

*½ tsp thyme*

Directions:

1.  Add onion, carrots, and celery into a slow cooker.

2.  Add stewing meat in a large bowl and season with pepper and salt.

3.  Add the almond flour and toss the meat until well coated.

4.  Fry the garlic in the hot oil for about one minute.

5.  Add the seasoned meat and all the flour from the bottom of the bowl to the pan.

6.  Cook the meat without stirring for a few minutes to allow it to brown on one side.

7.  Flip and repeat until all the sides of the beef are browned.

8.  Add the browned beef to the slow cooker and stir to combine with the vegetables.

9.  Add the beef stock, Dijon mustard, Worcestershire sauce, soyosauce, xylitol, thyme, and rosemary to the skillet.

10. Stir to combine all ingredients and dissolve the browned bits from the bottom of the skillet.

11. Once everything is dissolved then pour the sauce over the ingredients in the slow cooker.

12. Cover slow cooker with lid and cook on high for four hours.

13. After cooking, remove the lid and stir stew well and using dork shred the beef into pieces.

14. Taste the stew and adjust the seasoning.

*[Calories 275 | Total Fats 10g | Net Carbs: 24g | Protein 22g]*

## The Best Browned Beef Stew

[Total Time: 6 HR 50 MIN| Serve: 8]

*Ingredients:*

*2.2 lbs beef stewing meat, (cut into bite-sized pieces)*

*1 tsp Salt*

*1 tsp pepper*

*1 medium onion, finely chopped*

*2 celery ribs, sliced*

*2-3 cloves of garlic, minced*

*1 canned tomato paste*

*1-liter beef stock*

*2 Tbsp Worcestershire sauce*

*2 cups frozen vegetables*

*¼ cup almond flour*

*¼ cup water*

Directions:

1. Combine beef, celery, carrots, red onion, potatoes, salt, pepper, garlic, parsley, oregano, Worcestershire sauce, beef broth, and tomato paste in the crock pot.

2. Cook on low for 10 hours or on HIGH for 6-7 hours.

3.  Just 30 minutes before serving, combine together flour and water in small bowl and pour into the crockpot.
4.  Stir until well combined.
5.  Add frozen vegetables and continue cooking covered for 30 minutes.

    *[Calories 173 | Total Fats 4g | Net Carbs: 20g | Protein 17g]*

## Thai Nut Chicken
[Total Time: 5 HR 15 MIN| Serve: 8]

*Ingredients:*

*8 boneless skinless chicken thighs (about 2 pounds)*

*½ cup coconut flour*

*3/4 cup creamy nut butter*

*½ cup orange juice*

*¼ cup diabetic apricot jam*

*2 tbsp sesame oil*

*2 tbsp soy sauce*

*2 tbsp teriyaki sauce*

*2 tbsp hoisin sauce*

*1 canned coconut milk*

*3/4 cup water*

*1 cup chopped roasted almonds or any of the other nuts on green list*

Directions:

1. Place coconut flour in a large re-sealable plastic bag.

2. Add chicken, a few pieces at a time, and shake to coat.

3. Transfer to a greased slow cooker.

4. In a small bowl, combine the nut butter, orange juice, jam, oil, soy sauce, teriyaki sauce, hoisin sauce and 3/4 cup coconut milk; pour over chicken. Cover and cook on low for 4-5 hours or until chicken is tender.

5. Sprinkle with nuts before serving.

*[Calories 363 | Total Fats 18.15g | Net Carbs: 11.6g | Protein 38.7g]*


## *Bouillabaisse Fish Stew*
[Total Time: 6 HR 55 MIN| Serve: 6]

*Ingredients:*

*1 cup dry white wine*

*juice and zest of 1 orange*

*2 tbsp olive oil*

*1 large onion, diced*

*2 cloves garlic, minced*

*1 tsp dried basil*

*1/2 tsp dried thyme*

*1/2 tsp salt*

*1/4 tsp ground black pepper*

*4 cups fish stock; chicken stock can also be used*

*1 can diced tomatoes, drained*

*1 bay leaf*

*0.9 lb boneless, skinless white fish fillet (ex. cod)*

*0.9 lb prawns peeled and deveined*

*0.9 lb mussels in their shells*

*Juice of ½ lemon*

*1/4 cup fresh Italian (flat-leaf) parsley*

Directions:

1.  Heat the oil in a large pan.
2.  Add the onion and fry all the vegetables until almost tender.
3.  Add the garlic, basil, thyme, salt, and pepper.
4.  Pour the wine and bring to a boil. Add the fish stock, orange zest, tomatoes, and bay leaf and stir to combine.
5.  Pour everything into a slow cooker, cover the cooker, and cook on low for 4 to 6 hours.
6.  About 30 minutes before serving, turn the cooker to high. Toss the fish and prawns with the lemon juice.
7.  Stir into the broth in the cooker, cover, and cook until the fish cooks through about 20 minutes.
8.  Add mussel's right at the end and allow to steam for 20 minutes with the lid on.

*[Calories 310 | Total Fats 30g | Net Carbs: 4g | Protein 3g]*

## Beef & Broccoli Stew

[Total Time: 2 HR 20 MIN| Serve: 8]

*Ingredients:*

*1 cup beef stock*

*¼ cup soy sauce*

*¼ cup oyster sauce*

*¼ cup Xylitol*

*1 tbsp sesame oil*

*3 cloves garlic, minced*

*2.2 lbs boneless beef chuck roast and thinly sliced*

*2 tbsp almond flour or psyllium husk*

*2 heads broccoli, cut into florets*

Directions:

1.  In a medium bowl, whisk together beef stock, soy sauce, oyster sauce, sugar, sesame oil, and garlic.

2.  Place beef into a slow cooker. Add sauce mixture and gently toss to combine. Cover and cook on low heat for 90 minutes.

3.  In a small bowl, whisk together 1/4 cup water and almond flour.

4.   Stir in almond flour mixture and broccoli into the slow cooker. Cover and cook on high heat for an additional 30 minutes.

   *[Calories 370 | Total Fats 18g | Net Carbs: 4g | Protein 47g]*

## Mussel Stew

[Total Time: 5 HR 45 MIN| Serve: 8]

*Ingredients:*

*2.2 lbs fresh or frozen, cleaned mussels*

*3 tbsp olive oil*

*4 cloves garlic, minced*

*1 Large onion, finely diced*

*1 punnet mushrooms, diced*

*2 cans diced tomatoes*

*2 tbsp oregano*

*½ tbsp basil*

*½ tsp black pepper*

*1 tsp paprika*

*Dash red chili flakes*

*3/4 cup water*

Directions:

1.   Fry onions, garlic, shallots and mushrooms, scrape entire contents of the pan into your crockpot.

2.  Add all remaining ingredients to your slow cooker except your mussels. Cook on low for 4-5 hours, or on high for 2-3 hours. You're cooking until your mushrooms are fork tender and until the flavors meld together.

3.  Once your mushrooms are cooked and your sauce is done, crank the crockpot up to high. Add cleaned mussels to the pot and secure lid tightly. Cook for 30 more minutes.

4.  Ladle your mussels into bowls with plenty of broth. If any mussels didn't open up during cooking, toss those as well.

    *[Calories 228 | Total Fats 9g | Net Carbs: 32g | Protein 4g]*

## Creamy Chicken & Pumpkin Stew
[Total Time: 5 HR| Serve: 6]

*Ingredients:*

*1.3 lb chicken boneless chicken breast*

*1 ¼ cups chicken stock*

*1 can evaporate milk (Full Cream)*

*1/3 cup of sour cream or crème Fraiche*

*1 tbsp minced garlic*

*½ cup grated mature cheddar cheese*

*Fresh or frozen finely chopped pumpkin*

*Salt and pepper to taste*

Directions:

1.  In a crockpot combine all ingredients.

2.  Cover and turn crock pot on low. Cook for 4.5 hours on low or until both chicken and pumpkin are cooked and soft.

3.  Stir sauce in crock pot prior to serving.

    *[Calories 321 | Total Fats 12g | Net Carbs: 17g | Protein 35g]*


## Sweet Potato Stew

[Total Time: 6 HR 20 MIN| Serve: 6]

*Ingredients:*

*2 cups cubed sweet potatoes*

*4 boneless chicken breasts*

*4 boneless chicken thighs*

*2 cups chicken stock*

*1 ½ cups chopped green sweet peppers*

*1 ¼ cup diced fresh tomatoes*

*¾ cup can tomatoes, onion and chili mix*

*1 tbsp Cajun or curry seasoning*

*2 cloves garlic, minced*

*¼ cup creamy nut*

*Fresh coriander*

*Chopped roasted nuts*

Directions:

1.  In a slow cooker sweet potatoes, chicken, broth, peppers, diced tomatoes, tomatoes and green chilies mix, Cajun seasoning, and garlic.

2.  Cover and cook on low-heat setting for 10 to 12 hours or on high-heat setting for 5 to 6 hours.

3.  Remove 1 cup hot liquid from cooker. Whisk the liquid with nut butter in a bowl. Add mixture in cooker.

4.  Serve topped with cilantro and, if desired, peanuts.

    *[Calories 399 | Total Fats 21g | Net Carbs: 13.5g | Protein 37g]*

## Oxtail Stew

[Total Time: 9 HR 15 MIN| Serve: 10]

*Ingredients:*

*3.3 lbs of oxtail*

*1 large pack grated cabbage*

*1 large pack grated carrots*

*2 large onions*

*1 large bunch of celery*

*1 tin of tomatoes*

*2 jelly stock cubes*

*2.5 liters of water*

*1 tbsp crushed garlic*

*1 branch rosemary*

*2 bay leaves*

Directions:

1.  Place all ingredients into a slow cooker and cook on medium for 9 hours.
2.  Season with salt and pepper
3.  Grate ½ cup cheddar cheese to finish (optional).
    *[Calories 152 | Total Fats 7g | Net Carbs: 5.4g | Protein 16.7g]*

# Italian Gnocchi Soup
[Total Time: 40 MIN| Serve: 6]

Ingredients:

*1.1 lbs ground spicy Italian sausage*

*1 small onion, diced*

*2 cloves garlic, minced*

*4 cups chicken stock or bone broth*

*1 red medium pepper, diced*

*1 cup chopped fresh or frozen spinach*

*½ cup heavy cream*

*Sea salt and freshly cracked black pepper*

*Optional garnish: Parmesan cheese, chopped parsley & crumbled bacon*

Directions:

1. Fry sausage, onion, and garlic. Cook until the sausage is completely browned. Stirring occasionally and break up the sausage with a spoon.

2. Add in the bone broth or chicken stock and diced red peppers to the pot and bring the mixture to a simmer.

3. Reduce heat to medium-low and add the spinach and cook for an additional 5 minutes

4. Add gnocchi & cream and stir to combine.

5. Season to taste with salt and pepper.

*[Calories 336 | Total Fats 17g | Net Carbs: 4.65g | Protein 40g]*

## Spanish Chorizo Soup
[Total Time: 12 HR 10 MIN| Serve: 6]

*Ingredients:*

*2 cups sweet potatoes, cubed and peeled*

*4 cups cabbage and carrot coleslaw mix*

*1 large onion, chopped*

*1.1 lbs chorizo halved lengthwise and cut into thick slices*

*4 cups chicken stock*

Directions:

1. Place potatoes, coleslaw mix, onion, caraway seeds and sausage in slow cooker. Pour stock into a pot.
2. Cover; cook on low for 10 - 12 hours or high for 5 - 6 hours.
3. You can also use beef, chicken, or pork sausages in place boerewors.

*[Calories 329 | Total Fats 12.4g | Net Carbs: 12g | Protein 40g]*

## Loaded Cauliflower Soup
[Total Time: 5 HR 15 MIN| Serve: 6]

*Ingredients:*

*3 cups cauliflower, chopped*

*1½ cups chicken stock*

*1½ cups water*

*¼ cup milk*

*¼ tsp salt*

*1 tbsp butter*

*3 cloves garlic, minced*

*3 tbsp parmesan*

*1 cup chopped onion*

*8-10 spring onions*

*Salt to taste*

*¼ tsp pepper*

*1 tbsp olive oil*

*½ tsp parsley*

*1 Packet of streaky bacon, chopped, fried crisp and crumbled*

*½ cup shredded cheddar cheese*

## Directions:

1. Chop cauliflower into chunks, add all ingredients to a slow cooker and cover and cook on low for 5 hours.

2. Ladle into bowls. Sprinkle with Parmesan cheese and parsley. (Optional: additional bacon, shredded cheese, and sour cream for topping)

   *[Calories 245 | Total Fats 14.3g | Net Carbs: 21g | Protein 11.7g]*

## *French Onion Soup*
## [Total Time: 8 HR 40 MIN| Serve: 8]

*Ingredients:*

*¼ cup unsalted butter*

*6 thyme sprigs*

*1 bay leaf*

*5 pounds large sweet onions, vertically sliced  (about 16 cups)*

*1 tbsp sugar*

*6 cups low-sodium beef stock*

*2 tbsp red wine vinegar*

*1 ½  tsp kosher salt*

*1 tsp black pepper*

*5 ounces Gruyere cheese, shredded  (about 1 ¼ cups)*

Directions:

1.  Place butter, thyme, and bay leaf in the bottom of a 6-quart slow cooker. Add onions; sprinkle with sugar. Cover and cook on high for 8 hours.
2.  Discard thyme and bay leaf.
3.  Add vinegar, stock, pepper and salt and stir well.
4.  Cover and cook, on HIGH for 30 minutes.

    *[Calories 258 | Total Fats 12.6g | Net Carbs: 10.8g | Protein 27g]*

## Thai Chicken Soup

[Total Time: 4 HR 15 MIN| Serve: 8]

*Ingredients:*

*2 tbsp red curry paste*

*2 cans of coconut milk*

*2 cups chicken stock*

*2 tbsp fish sauce*

*2 tbsp Xylitol*

*2 tbsp nut butter*

*6-8 chicken breasts cut into pieces*

*1 red bell pepper, seeded and sliced*

*1 onion, thinly sliced*

*4-6 large grated carrots*

*1 heaped tbsp fresh ginger, minced*

*1 tbsp lime juice*

*Coriander for garnish*

Directions:

1.  Mix the curry paste, coconut milk, chicken stock, fish sauce, Xylitol and nut butter in a slow-cooker bowl.
2.  Place the chicken breast, red bell pepper, onion, grated carrots and ginger in the slow cooker, cover and cook on high for 4 hours.
3.  Add in the mange tout at the end of the cooking time and cook for a ½ hour longer. Stir in lime juice and serve with coriander.

    *[Calories 258 | Total Fats 12.6g | Net Carbs: 10.8g | Protein 27g]*

## *Curried Cauliflower Soup*
[Total Time: 25 MIN| Serve: 6]

*Ingredients:*

*1 tbsp olive oil*

*1 medium spring onion*

*1 cup cauliflower, steamed*

*1 cup beef stock*

*½ cup coconut milk*

*10 cashew nuts*

*½ tsp coriander*

½ tsp turmeric

½ tsp cumin

2 tbsp fresh parsley, finely chopped

salt and pepper, to taste


Directions:

1. Place the cauliflower and onion in a large pot and add chicken stock. Stir in coriander, turmeric, cumin and a pinch of salt. Bring to a boil and let boil for 5 minutes.

2. Remove from heat. Using a hand blender, puree ingredients in the pot until smooth. Stir in the coconut milk. Serve with roasted cashew nuts and top with parsley.

   *[Calories 258 | Total Fats 12.6g | Net Carbs: 10.8g | Protein 27g]*


## *Easy Everyday Chicken Soup*
[Total Time: 5 HR| Serve: 8]

*Ingredients:*

*3 skinned, bone-in chicken breasts*

*6 skinned and boned chicken thighs*

*1 tsp salt*

*½ tsp freshly ground pepper*

*½ tsp chicken spice seasoning*

*3-4 carrots sliced*

*4 celery ribs, sliced*

*1 sweet onion, chopped*

*2 cans evaporated milk*

*2 cups chicken stock*

Directions:

1. Prepare Chicken: Rub chicken pieces with salt, pepper, and chicken spice seasoning. Place breasts in a slow cooker, top with thighs.

2. Add carrots and next 3 ingredients. Whisk evaporated milk and stock until smooth. Pour soup mixture over vegetables.

3. Cover with lid and cook on high 3 and half hours.

4. Remove chicken from slow cooker and allow to cool for 10 minutes.

5. Using fork shred the chicken.

6. Stir shredded chicken into the soup-and-vegetable mixture.

7. Cover again with lid and cook on HIGH for 1 hour.

   *[Calories 282 | Total Fats 18g | Net Carbs: 5.6g | Protein 24g]*

## *Creamy Chicken & Tomato Soup*
[Total Time: 9 HR 10 MIN| Serve: 8]

*Ingredients:*

*8 frozen skinless boneless chicken breast*

*2 tbsp Italian Seasoning*

*1 tbsp dried basil*

*2 cloves garlic, minced*

*1 large onion, chopped*

*2 can of coconut milk (full fat), shake before opening can avoid separation*

*2 cans diced tomatoes and juice*

*2 ¼ cups of chicken stock*

*1 small can of tomato paste*

*Sea salt and pepper to taste*

Directions:

1. Put all the above ingredients into the slow cooker, cook for 9 hours on low.

2. After 9 hours take two forks and shred the chicken, set the slow cooker on warm till ready to serve

   *[Calories 227 | Total Fats 3.8g | Net Carbs: 6.37g | Protein 30g]*

## Tomato & Basil Soup

[Total Time: 7 HR 45 MIN| Serve: 6]

*Ingredients:*

*2 cans diced tomatoes, with juice*

*1 cup finely diced celery*

*1 cup finely diced carrots*

*1 cup finely diced onions*

*1 tsp dried oregano or 1 T fresh oregano*

*1 tbsp dried basil or ¼ cup fresh basil*

*4 cups chicken stock*

*½ tsp bay leaf*

*1 cup Parmesan cheese*

*½ cup butter*

*2 cups full cream milk*

*1 tsp salt*

*¼ tsp black pepper*

*¼ cup almond flour or ground chia seeds*

Directions:

1. Add tomatoes, celery, carrots, chicken stock, onions, oregano, basil, and bay leaf to a large slow cooker.

2. Cover and cook on low for 5-7 hours, until flavors, are blended and vegetables are tender.

3. About 30 minutes before serving, Melt butter over low heat and add almond flour. Stir constantly with a whisk for 5-7 minutes.

4. Slowly stir in 1 cup hot soup. Add another 3 cups and stir until smooth. Add all back into the slow cooker.

5. Stir and add the Parmesan cheese, milk, salt, and pepper.

6. Cover and cook on LOW for another 30 minutes or so until ready to serve.

*[Calories 269 | Total Fats 11g | Net Carbs: 4.86g | Protein 35.71g]*

## Beef & Cabbage Soup

[Total Time: 8 HR 15 MIN| Serve: 8]

Ingredients:

*2 tbsp olive or coconut oil*

*1.1 lbs ground beef mince*

*½ large onion, chopped*

*5 cups chopped cabbage*

*2 cups water*

*2 tins tomato puree*

*4 beef stock cubes*

*1 ½ tsp ground cumin*

*1 tsp salt*

*1 tsp pepper*

Directions:

1.  Heat oil in a large pot.
2.  Add ground beef and onion, and cook until beef brown and crumbled.
3.  Transfer mince with fat to a slow cooker. Add cabbage, water, tomato sauce, bouillon, cumin, salt, and pepper. Stir to dissolve stock cubes and cover.

4.  Cook on high setting for 4 hours, or on low setting for 6 to 8 hours. Stir occasionally.

    *[Calories 165 | Total Fats 8g | Net Carbs: 13.7g | Protein 11.54g]*


# Vegetable Beef Soup

[Total Time: 8 HR 45 MIN| Serve: 4]

*Ingredients:*

*1.1 lbs ground beef mince*

*2 cups tomato-vegetable juice cocktail*

*2 packages frozen mixed vegetables*


Directions:

1.  Place ground beef mince in a slow cooker. Cook over medium-high heat until evenly brown and crumble.
2.  Add juice cocktail and mixed vegetables.
3.  In a slow cooker oven, simmer for 30 minutes.
4.  In a slow cooker, cook 1 hour on High.
5.  Then reduce heat to Low and simmer 6 to 8 hours.

    *[Calories 251 | Total Fats 12g | Net Carbs: 13.5g | Protein 21.3g]*


# Clam Chowder

[Total Time: 11 HR 15 MIN| Serve: 8]

*Ingredients:*

*2 can minced clams in brine*

*4 slices bacon, cut into small pieces*

*3 sweet potatoes, peeled and cubed*

*1 cup chopped onion*

*1 carrot, grated*

*1 punnet mushrooms fried in butter and blended finely with a hand blender*

*¼ tsp ground black pepper*

*2 cans evaporated milk*

Directions:

1. In a small bowl, drain the clams and reserve the juice.

2. Add water to the juice as needed to total 1 3/4 cups liquid. Cover the clams and put in refrigerator for later.

3. In a slow cooker combine the bacon, sweet potatoes, onion, carrot, mushrooms, ground black pepper, evaporated milk and reserved clam juice with water.

4. Cover and cook on low setting for 9 to 11 hours or on high setting for 4 to 5 hours. Add the clams and cook on high setting for another hour.

   *[Calories 206 | Total Fats 9.56g | Net Carbs: 21.42g | Protein 9.24g]*

# Mushroom Soup

[Total Time: 6 HR 55 MIN| Serve: 8]

*Ingredients:*

*2 punnets white button mushrooms, cleaned, trimmed, and quartered*

*1 medium onion, roughly chopped*

*4 cloves garlic, sliced*

*7 sprigs thyme, divided*

*2 small lemons, halved*

*2 tbsp olive oil*

*1 ½ tbsp red wine vinegar*

*Salt and freshly ground black pepper*

*½ cup dry sherry*

*2 cups milk*

*1 cup heavy cream*

*½ cup sour cream*

*3 cups chicken stock or vegetable stock*

Directions:

1.  Preheat oven to 375ºF.

2.  Place mushrooms, onions, garlic, and 5 thyme sprigs in a large bowl. Squeeze lemons into the bowl and add the squeezed lemon halves. Add vinegar and olive oil.

3.  Season with salt and pepper and toss to coat.

4.  Transfer to a foil-lined rimmed baking sheet and spread into an even layer.

5.  Roast in preheated oven until mushrooms release liquid, about 15 minutes.

6.  Carefully drain liquid into a separate container and reserve.

7.  Return mushrooms to oven and continue roasting until browned about 30 minutes.

8.  Discard lemons and thyme sprigs.

9.  Transfer mushroom mixture along with drained liquid to the slow cooker.

10. Add milk, heavy cream, sour cream, sherry, and stock, along with remaining thyme sprigs. Stir well.

11. Cook on low for 6 hours.

12. Discard thyme sprigs.

13. Transfer soup to a blender and blend until you get desiredoconsistency.

*[Calories 198 | Total Fats 13.2g | Net Carbs: 15.8g | Protein 5g]*

## Seafood Soup

[Total Time: 4 HR 15 MIN| Serve: 8]

*Ingredients:*

*12 slices bacon, chopped*

*2 cloves garlic, minced*

*6 cups chicken stock*

*3 stalks celery, diced*

*2 large carrots, diced*

Ground black pepper to taste

½ tsp red pepper flakes, or to taste

2 cups onions

2 cup uncooked prawns, peeled and deveined

1.1 lbs white fish fillets like Hake or Kingklip, cut into bite-size pieces

1 can evaporate milk


Directions:

1. Fry bacon in coconut oil or olive oil, add onion and garlic. Transfer mixture to a slow cooker.

2. Pour chicken stock into slow cooker. Add celery, and carrots into the stock. Season with black pepper and red pepper flakes.

3. Set the cooker to high, cover, and cook for 3 hours.

4. Stir prawns and fish into the soup and cook 1 more hour. Stir evaporated milk into chowder, heat thoroughly, and serve.

*[Calories 281 | Total Fats 9.5g | Net Carbs: 7.8g | Protein 39g]*


## Cream of Broccoli 'n' Mushroom Soup
[Total Time: 4 HR 15 MIN| Serve: 6]

*Ingredients:*

*1 tbsp oil*

*1 onion, chopped*

*2 packets frozen chopped broccoli, thawed*

2 cans cream of celery soup

2 punnets of mushrooms fried in butter and blitzed smooth with a hand blender

1 cup shredded cheddar cheese

2 cans evaporated milk

Directions:

1.  Fry the onion in coconut oil and transfer to the slow cooker.

2.  Transfer the drained onion to a slow cooker.

3.  Place the broccoli, cream of celery soup, mushrooms, cheddar cheese, and milk into the slow cooker.

4.  Cook on low for 3-4 hours or until the broccoli is tender.

    *[Calories 212 | Total Fats 4.7g | Net Carbs: 36.6g | Protein 10g]*

## Beef 'n' Vegetable Soup

[Total Time: 8 HR 15 MIN| Serve: 8]

*Ingredients:*

*2.2 lbs beef chuck or neck*

*1 can diced tomatoes, undrained*

*2 medium sweet potatoes, peeled and cubed*

*2 medium onions, diced*

*3 celery ribs, sliced*

*2 carrots, sliced*

*2 cups pumpkin*

*3 beef stock cubes*

*½ tsp salt*

*½ tsp dried basil*

*½ tsp dried oregano*

*¼ tsp pepper*

*3 cups water*

Directions:

1.  In a slow cooker, combine all the ingredients. Cover and cook on high for 6-8 hours

    *[Calories 253 | Total Fats 14.5g | Net Carbs: 10g | Protein 23g]*

## Cream of Carrot Soup
[Total Time: 8 HR 25 MIN| Serve: 6]

*Ingredients:*

*1 onion, diced*

*2 stalks celery, diced*

*1 large sweet potato, diced*

*8 whole carrots, sliced*

*4 cups chicken broth stock*

*1 whole bay leaf*

*Salt and pepper, to taste*

*4 dashes Tabasco (or other hot sauce)*

*1 cup heavy cream*

1 tsp parsley

Directions:

1.  Add all ingredients except parsley and heavy cream to a slow cooker.

2.  Cover and cook on low for 6-8 hours.

3.  Discard bay leaf.

4.  Using a hand blender, puree the vegetables.

5.  Turn heat to high and stir in parsley and heavy cream.

6.  Cook for another 15 minutes to allow the heavy cream to heat thoroughly.

    *[Calories 356 | Total Fats 31.7g | Net Carbs: 14.7g | Protein 5g]*

## Cream of Tomato Soup

[Total Time: 6 HR 15 MIN| Serve: 6]

*Ingredients:*

*2 tbsp unsalted butter*

*2 large onion, finely chopped*

*2 cans diced tomatoes with juice*

*1 cup chicken stock*

*1 cup heavy cream, warmed*

*¼ tsp cayenne pepper*

*Salt and pepper to taste*

Directions:

1. Melt butter and fry the onion in it. Transfer to slow cooker.
2. Add tomatoes with juice, half cup water, and stock into the cooker and stir well.
3. Cover with lid and cook on low for 5 to 6 hours.
4. Puree the soup with a blender, then stir in cream.
5. Season with pepper and salt.
6. Serve and enjoy.

   *[Calories 229 | Total Fats 11.5g | Net Carbs: 6g | Protein 24.9g]*

## *Creamy Zucchini Soup*

[Total Time: 2 HR 20 MIN| Serve: 6]

*Ingredients:*

*1 small onion, minced*

*4 cups grated zucchini with peel*

*2 cups chicken stock*

*1 tsp salt*

*1 tsp dried dill*

*½ tsp white pepper*

*2 tbsp butter, melted*

*1 cup sour cream*

Directions:

1.  Mix together everything except the sour cream in a greased slow cooker.

2.  Cook covered for 2 hours on low.

3.  Mix in the sour cream and cook for an additional 10 minutes, or until heated through.

*[Calories 233 | Total Fats 8.5g | Net Carbs: 3.41g | Protein 34g]*

## Indian Curried Cauliflower Soup
[Total Time: 5 HR 15 MIN| Serve: 4]

*Ingredients:*

*1 head cauliflower*

*2 cups chicken stock*

*3 cloves garlic*

*1 canned coconut milk*

*1 cup plain yogurt*

*1 tbsp curry powder*

*Salt and pepper to taste*

*¼ cup toasted pine nuts*

*¾ tsp garam masala*

*½ cup xylitol*

½ tsp salt

1 tbsp water

Directions:

1.  Cut cauliflower from the stalk, place in slow cooker, put chicken stock and garlic in the slow cooker.

2.  Cover and cook until tender, about 2-4 hours on low.

3.  Add coconut milk and yogurt to slow cooker and cook for an additional 1 hour on low, then using a hand blender.

4.  Blend until pureed.

5.  Sprinkle with toasted pine nuts and some fresh mint.

    *[Calories 219 | Total Fats 7g | Net Carbs: 4.13g | Protein 33.7g]*

## Broccoli 'n' Blue cheese Soup
[Total Time: 4 HR 20 MIN| Serve: 6]

*Ingredients:*

*2 onion, diced*

*4 stick celery, sliced*

*4 leek, sliced (white part only)*

*2 tbsp butter*

*4 cups chicken stock*

*2 large heads of broccoli, cut into florets*

*1 ¼ cups crumbled blue cheese*

½ *cup cream*

Directions:

1.  Put all of the ingredients into your slow cooker.

2.  Stir to combine.

3.  Put the lid on the slow cooker and cook on high for 4 hours (or 8 hours on low).

4.  Using a hand blender, blitz the soup until smooth Ladle into bowls and top with extra crumbles of blue cheese (if desired).

    *[Calories 174 | Total Fats 10g | Net Carbs: 12.8g | Protein 7.5g]*


## Italian Meatball Zoodle Soup
[Total Time: 6 HR 45 MIN| Serve: 6]

*Ingredients:*

*32 oz. beef stock*

*1 medium zucchini, spiraled*

*2 ribs celery, chopped*

*1 small onion, diced*

*1 carrot, chopped*

*1 medium tomato, diced*

*1 ½ tsp garlic salt*

*1 ½ lb. ground beef*

*½ cup parmesan cheese, shredded*

*6 cloves garlic, minced*

1 egg

4 Tbsp fresh parsley, chopped

1 ½ tsp sea salt

1 ½ tsp onion powder

1 tsp Italian seasoning

1 tsp dried oregano

½ tsp black pepper

Directions:

1. Heat slow cooker on low setting.

2. Add zucchini, celery, tomato, carrot onion, beef stock and garlic salt into the slow cooker. Cover.

3. In a large bowl, combine together Italian seasoning, oregano, onion powder, sea salt, parsley, egg, garlic, parmesan, ground beef, and pepper.

4. Using mixture make approximately 30 meatballs.

5. Heat olive oil in a large skillet over medium-high heat.

6. Once the pan is hot, add meatballs and brown on all sides.

7. Add meatballs into the slow cooker, cover with a lid and cook for 6 hours.

*[Calories 352 | Total Fats 19g | Net Carbs: 4.5g | Protein 40g]*

## BBQ Chicken Soup

[Total Time: 1 HR 50 MIN| Serve: 4]

*Ingredients:*

*For Soup Base:*

*3 chicken thighs*

*Salt*

*1 ½ cups chicken broth*

*2 tsp chili seasoning*

*2 tbsp olive oil*

*1 ½ cups beef broth*

*Black pepper*

*For BBQ Sauce:*

*¼ cup ketchup*

*2 tbsp Dijon mustard*

*1 tbsp hot sauce*

*1 tsp Worcestershire sauce*

*1 tsp onion powder*

*1 tsp red chili flakes*

*¼ cup butter*

*¼ cup tomato paste*

*1 tbsp soy sauce*

*2 ½ tsp liquid smokes*

*1 ½ tsp garlic powder*

*1 tsp chili powder*

*1 tsp cumin*

## Directions:

1. Set oven to 400⁰F. Remove bones from chicken and put bones aside. Season chicken with chili seasoning and place into oven for 50 minutes.

2. Heat oil in a deep pot and add bones. Cook for 5 minutes then add beef and chicken broth; season with pepper and salt.

3. Take chicken from oven and remove skin. Add the fat to the soup and mix together. Combine BBQ sauce ingredients and add to pot. Cook for 30 minutes.

4. Combine fats in the soup by using an immersion blender then shred chicken and add to soup. Cook for 20 minutes.

5. Serve topped with chicken skin. May add cheese or bell peppers.

   *[Calories 487 | Total Fats 38.3g | Net Carbs: 4.3g | Protein 24.5g | Fiber: 1.3g]*

## *Super-Fast Egg Drop Soup*

[Total Time: 15 MIN| Serve: 1]

*Ingredients:*

*1 ½ cups chicken broth*

*1 tbsp butter*

*1 tsp chili garlic paste*

*½ cube chicken bouillon*

*2 eggs*

Directions:

1.  Add butter to pan, heat until it melts then add broth and bouillon

2.  Bring to a boil and add chili paste, stir to combine and remove from flame.

3.  Beat eggs in a bowl and add to broth, stir and put aside for a few minutes.

4.  Serve.

    *[Calories 279 | Total Fats 23g | Net Carbs: 2.5g | Protein 12g]*

## Spicy Slow-Cooked Chicken Soup
[Total Time: 6 HR 10 MIN| Serve: 4]

*Ingredients:*

*4 pcs boneless chicken fillet*

*4 bacon strips*

*1 small onion, sliced thin*

*1 bell pepper, sliced thin*

*½ tbsp fresh thyme*

*½ tbsp garlic, minced*

*½ tbsp coconut flour*

*½ cup low-sodium chicken stock*

*¼ cup coconut milk, unsweetened*

1 ½ tbsp tomato paste

1 ½ tbsp lemon juice

1 tbsp butter

Salt and pepper to taste

Directions:

1.  Place the butter in the middle of the slow cooker.

2.  Add the onion and bell pepper slices at the bottom and then top with the chicken fillet

3.  Chop the bacon and sprinkle on top of the chicken.

4.  Add the rest of the ingredients (liquids last) and then cover and cook on low for 6 hours.

5.  Uncover after 6 hours and break the chicken before serving.

6.  Serve with a spoon full of sour cream on top.

    *(Calories 396 | Total Fats 21g | Net Carbs: 7g | Protein 41g | Fiber: 2g)*

## BBQ Pizza Soup

[Total Time: 25 MIN| Serve: 8]

Ingredients:

6 Chicken legs

4 Garlic Cloves

4 Cups Green beans

1 ½ cups Mozzarella cheese

*3 Liters Water*

*½ Tsp Black pepper*

*1 Red Onion (chopped)*

*14 oz. canned tomatoes (sugar-free)*

*¾ Cup BBQ sauce*

*¼ cup Ghee*

*1 tsp Salt*

*Basil (chopped)*

Directions:

1. Add water and salt to a pot and boil chicken for 60 minutes or more until meat is falling off bones. Shred chicken and put aside until needed.

2. Heat ghee in a soup pot and sauté garlic and onion until golden and aromatic. Add broth from boiling chicken by straining into the pot.

3. Clean and chop beans and add to pot along with tomatoes. Cook for 15 minutes.

4. Add shredded chicken and BBQ sauce and remove from flame. Add pepper and salt to taste.

5. Top with mozzarella cheese, stir and ladle into bowls.

6. Serve topped with basil.

*[Calories 449 | Total Fats 32.5g | Net Carbs: 10g | Protein 30.8g | Fiber 2.8g]*

# Cheese and Bacon Soup

[Total Time: 30 MIN| Serve: 4]

*Ingredients:*

*3 bacon strips, cooked and chopped*

*1 cup cheddar, shredded*

*1 cup Monterey jack cheese, shredded*

*1 small bell pepper, chopped*

*2 cloves of garlic, minced*

*1 onion, chopped fine*

*12 oz. gluten-free beer*

*½ cup milk*

*½ cup light cream*

*2 tbsp butter*

*2 tbsp flour*

*Salt and pepper to taste*

Directions:

1. Using the grease from cooking bacon, sauté the onions and bell pepper for 5 minutes in a pot over medium heat.

2. Adjust the heat to low and add the garlic and cook for another 2 minutes.

3. Increase the heat again and then add the 2 tbsp butter and allow it to boil.

4. Add the 2 tbsp flour to the pot and whisk for 3 minutes.

5. Pour the beer and stir constantly for 5 minutes.

6. Lower the heat again and add the milk and light cream.

7. Remove the pot from the head and then add the cheese. Stir until the cheese has completely melted.

8. Season with salt and pepper and transfer into serving bowls.

9. Garnish with crispy bacon on top. Serve hot.

*[Calories 442 | Total Fats 34g | Net Carbs: 11g | Protein 20g]*

## Beef Cabbage Parsley Soup
[Total Time: 2 HR 5 MIN| Serve: 8]

*Ingredients:*

*1 lb. beef shank*

*½ head cabbage, chopped*

*6 tsp fresh parsley (chopped)*

*2 zucchini, cubed*

*1 tomato, quartered*

*1 onion, chopped*

*4 cloves garlic, minced*

*1 Tbsp salt*

*¼ tsp ground cumin*

*2 Tbsp fresh lime juice*

Directions:

1.  In a large pot over low heat combine the beef, tomato, zucchini, onion, cabbage, garlic, 5 tsp parsley, salt, and cumin.

2.  Add water to cover and stir well. Cover the lid and cook for 2 hours.

3.  Remove lid, stir, and simmer for another 1 hour with lid off.

4.  Just before eating, squeeze in fresh lime juice to taste and sprinkle with remaining parsley.

5.  Serve hot.

    *[Calories 129 | Total Fats 2.3g | Net Carbs: 13.2g | Protein 14.1g | Fiber 2g]*

## *Boneless Lamb Stew*

[Total Time: 2 HR 10 MIN| Serve: 6]

*Ingredients:*

*2 lbs. boneless lamb meat, cubed*

*1 cup red onion, chopped*

*2 whole celery stalks, diced*

*4 cloves garlic, minced*

*1 cup tomato juice*

*2 Tbsp extra virgin coconut oil*

*1 cup lime juice (freshly squeezed)*

*1 bay leaf*

*1 tsp ground cinnamon*

*1 tsp ground nutmeg*

*Fresh parsley, chopped for topping*

*Sea salt and freshly ground black pepper, to taste*

Directions:

1. Put the lamb in a glass bowl and season with the salt, pepper, cinnamon, and nutmeg. Place in refrigerator for up to 24 hours.

2. In a large casserole, heat the coconut oil over medium heat. Add pieces of lamb and brown on all sides.

3. Once browned, add the onion, garlic, and celery. Cook for about five minutes, stirring often until vegetables start to soften.

4. Add the tomato juice, lime juice, and bay leaf; stir till mixture begins to boil.

5. Reduce the heat to low and cook for about 2 hours.

6. Serve hot with fresh chopped parsley.

*[Calories 250 | Total Fats 11.8g | Net Carbs: 6.8g | Protein 21g | Fiber 1.6g]*

## Keto Butternut Squash Soup

[Total Time: 55 MIN| Serve: 10]

*Ingredients:*

*3 lbs. butternut squash*

*4 cloves garlic, minced*

*1 cup yellow onion, sliced*

*1 cup coconut milk*

*2 tsp olive oil*

*1 bay leaf*

*2 cup water*

*½ tsp salt and pepper (per taste)*

*Coconut oil or olive oil for greasing*

Directions:

1. Preheat oven to 450$^0$F.

2. On a greased baking sheet, place the squash and onion with half oil and salt. Roast in a single layer about 25-30 minutes.

3. Transfer the vegetables to a large saucepan with olive oil and cook over HIGH heat for 3-5 minutes. Stir often.

4. Add garlic and cook for another 30 seconds. Add the water, bay leaf, and coconut milk; bring to a boil.

5. Reduce heat to MEDIUM-LOW, cover and simmer for 10 minutes more.

6. At the end, remove bay leaf and transfer squash mixture to a blender. Puree until smooth. Add salt and pepper to taste.

7. Ladle into bowls and serve hot.

*[Calories 120 | Total Fats 7.2g | Net Carbs: 12.7g | Protein 3.4g | Fiber: 2.3 g]*

## Spinach Soup with Almonds 'n' Parmesan

[Total Time: 45 MIN| Serve: 6]

*Ingredients:*

*1 lb. baby spinach leaves*

*1 leek*

*1 zucchini (medium)*

*¼ cup parmesan cheese (grated)*

*4 Tbsp olive oil*

*4 cups water*

*15 almond shivers*

*Salt and black ground pepper to taste*

Directions:

1. Wash the leek and cut it into thick slices.

2. Heat the olive oil in a saucepan and cook the zucchini and leek for about 2-3 minutes.

3. Add the cleaned spinach leaves, water and a pinch of salt. Bring to the boil and let it simmer for 15 minutes.

4. Remove from the heat and place the vegetables in a food processor. Blend into a very smooth soup.

5. In a frying pan, toast the almonds. Pour the soup into bowls, sprinkle with some Parmesan cheese on top and toasted almonds.

6. Serve.

   *[Calories 63.4 | Total Fats 3.4g | Net Carbs: 5.9g | Protein 4.84g | Fiber: 2.4g]*

## *Keto Light Cabbage Soup*
[Total Time: 35 MIN| Serve: 4]

*Ingredients:*

*2 ½ cups chopped cabbage*

*4 garlic cloves, minced*

*1 Tbsp tomato paste*

*1 onion, chopped*

*½ cup parsnip, chopped*

½ cup cauliflower florets

½ cup chopped zucchini

½ tsp basil

½ tsp oregano

Salt and black pepper, to taste

4 cups water

Olive oil for sautéing


Directions:

1.  In a frying pan, sauté onions, parsnip, and garlic for 5 minutes.
2.  Add in water, tomato paste, cabbage, cauliflower, basil, oregano and salt and pepper to taste.
3.  Simmer for about 5-10 minutes until all vegetables are tender. Add the zucchini and simmer for another 5 minutes.
4.  Serve hot.

    *[Calories 80.31| Total Fats 3.8g | Net Carbs: 9.69g | Protein 4.62g | Fiber: 1.6g]*


## Oriental Shrimp Soup
[Total Time: 25 MIN| Serve: 8]

*Ingredients:*

*12 oz. fresh shrimp, peeled and deveined*

*1 cup zucchini (medium, sliced)*

1 onion, chopped

2 cloves garlic, minced

1 Tbsp ginger, minced

1 pinch crushed red pepper

2 quarts water

1 cup celery (chopped)

2 cups cauliflower florets

2 Tbsp soy sauce

¼ tsp ground black pepper

2 tsp olive oil

Directions:

1.  In a large saucepan with over medium heat cook onion, garlic, ginger and crushed red pepper for 2 minutes.

2.  Pour in water, cauliflower florets, and celery and bring to a boil. Reduce heat, cover and simmer 5 minutes.

3.  Stir in zucchini and shrimp, season with salt and pepper to taste; cover and cook 5 - 7 minutes.

4.  Stir in soy sauce and pepper and serve.
    *[Calories 107.62 | Total Fats 3.08g | Net Carbs: 7.12g | Protein 12.08g | Fiber: 1.6g]*

### Zucchini Soup with Crunchy Cured Ham
[Total Time: 45 MIN| Serve: 4]

Ingredients:

*2 leeks  (white part only)*

*12 ounces zucchini*

*10 ounces summer squash*

*3 Tbsp extra virgin olive oil*

*5 cups water*

*Salt*

*2 slices cured ham*

*Black pepper*

Directions:

1.  Cut the leeks into thin slices and chop the zucchini and summer squash into cubes.

2.  In a large saucepan, heat the olive oil and add the leeks. Cook the leeks until they are soft, stirring gently.

3.  Add in the chopped zucchini and summer squash and cook them for about 5 minutes.

4.  Add in water and bring to the boil for about 15 minutes.

5.  Blend or process the soup in batches until smooth.

6.  Season the soup to taste.

7.  In a frying pan cook striped ham until crispy.

8.  Divide the soup amongst the serving bowls and sprinkle with the crunchy ham strips and some black pepper.

9.  Serve hot.

    *[Calories 84.19 | Total Fats 31.7g | Net Carbs: 8.75g | Protein 854g | Fiber: 1.52g]*

## Hot Chili Soup

[Total Time: 45 MIN| Serve: 4]

*Ingredients:*

*1 tsp Coriander seeds*

*2 Chili pepper, sliced*

*2 cups Water*

*½ tsp Ground cumin*

*16 oz Chicken thighs*

*1 Avocado*

*4 tbsp Cilantro, chopped*

*Salt*

*2 tbsp Olive oil*

*2 cups Chicken broth*

*1 tsp Turmeric*

*4 tbsp Tomato paste*

*2 tbsp Butter*

*2 oz Queso Fresco*

*Lime juice freshly squeezed*

*Black pepper*

Directions:

1. Chop chicken thighs and heat oil in a soup pot. Add chicken to the pot and cook for 8 minutes then remove from pot and put aside.

2. Add coriander to the pot and cook until aromatic then add chili and cook for 1 minute.

3. Add water and broth and bring mixture to a boil. Add cumin, turmeric, black pepper and salt to taste.

4. When soup starts to boil add butter and tomato paste, stir until butter melts and the mixture is thoroughly combined. Cook for 10 minutes then adds lime juice.

5. Add cooked chicken to soup and cook for 5 minutes.

6. Serve topped with queso fresco and avocado.

   *[Calories 396 | Total Fats 27.8g | Net Carbs: 5.8g | Protein 28g | Fiber: 5g]*


## Jalapeno Popper Soup
[Total Time: 1 HR 30 MIN| Serve: 6]

*Ingredients:*

*Salt*

*Black pepper*

*3 Jalapenos, diced*

*1 tsp Onion powder*

*1 tsp Cajun seasoning*

*3 cups Chicken broth*

*4 oz Cheddar cheese*

*4 Chicken thighs, bones removed*

*1 tbsp Chicken fat*

*2 tsp Garlic, diced*

*1 tsp Cilantro, dried*

*6 oz Cream cheese*

*4 Bacon slices*

Directions:

1. Set oven to 400⁰F.
2. Remove bones from thighs, season with pepper and salt and bake for 55 minutes.
3. Heat pot and heat 1 tbsp chicken fat then add bones to pot; fry for 10 minutes.
4. Add garlic and jalapeno, cook for 4 minutes until vegetables are softened.
5. Add spice to pot, stir and add broth, scraping pan to remove bits and cook until chicken is thoroughly cooked. Take skins from thighs and take bones from broth.
6. Add remaining fat to the pot along with garlic and jalapenos and use an immersion blender to puree mixture. Shred chicken and put into the pot, cook

for 15 minutes then add cheddar and cream cheese. Cook for 5 minutes until cheese melts.

7. Heat skillet and cook bacon until crisp. Cool and crumble bacon.

8. Serve soup with bacon on top and chickenoskins.

   *[Calories 550 | Total Fats 42.7g | Net Carbs: 3g | Protein 33.7g | Fiber 0.2g]*

## Cheeseburger Soup

[Total Time: 40 MIN| Serve: 5]

*Ingredients:*

*12 oz Ground beef*

*3 cups Beef broth*

*½ tsp Onion powder*

*1 ½ tsp kosher salt*

*½ tsp Red pepper flakes*

*1 tsp Chili powder*

*1 Dill pickle, diced*

*3 oz Cream cheese*

*5 Bacon slices*

*2 tbsp Butter*

*½ tsp Garlic powder*

*2 tsp Brown mustard*

*½ tsp Black pepper*

*1 tsp Cumin*

*2 ½ tbsp Tomato paste*

*1 cup Cheddar cheese, shredded*

*½ cup Heavy cream*

Directions:

1.  Heat pan and cook bacon until crisp, remove from pot and put aside until needed.

2.  Add beef to pot and cook for 10 minutes until browned all over.

3.  Transfer beef to a soup pot, add butter to the soup pot along with spices and cook for 45 seconds. Then add tomato paste, pickles, beef broth and cheese, cook for 3 minutes until melted.

4.  Lower heat and cook for 30 minutes.

5.  Remove from heat and add bacon and cream stir and

6.  serve.

    *[Calories 572 | Total Fats 48.6g | Net Carbs: 3.4g | Protein 23.4g | Fiber: 0.8g]*

## *Malaysian Bone Broth Soup*

[Total Time: 1 HR 10 MIN| Serve: 5]

*Ingredients:*

*2 lb pork ribs, cut into cubes*

*1 whole garlic, crushed*

1 cup dried shiitake mushrooms

1 cup enoki mushrooms

2 sachets Bak Kuh Teh

Pepper to taste

12 cups water

Directions:

1. Bring the water to a boil with the Bak Kuh Teh sachets in it.

2. When boiling, place the ribs in the pot and reduce the heat.

3. Throw the crushed garlic into the pot and then add the mushrooms. Stir.

4. Cook for 1 hour or a few minutes more.

5. Serve hot.

   [Calories 517 | Total Fats 32.2g | Net Carbs: 5.0g | Protein 48.8g | Fiber 1.0 g]

## Cheeseburger Soup Indulgence

[Total Time: 40 MIN| Serve: 5]

Ingredients:

5 strips of bacon, cooked and crumbled

12 oz ground beef

3 cups beef broth

2 tbsp organic butter

½ tsp onion powder

½ tsp garlic powder

2 tsp Dijon mustard

1 ½ tsp salt

½ tsp pepper

½ tsp red pepper flakes

1 tsp cumin

1 tsp chili powder

2 ½ tbsp tomato paste

¼ cup pickles, diced

1 cup cheddar cheese, shredded

¼ cream cheese

½ cup heavy cream

Directions:

1.  Using the same pan where the bacon was cooked, add the ground beef and cook until done.
2.  Place the browned beef into a pot and add the butter and the spices. Cook for 45 seconds.
3.  Pour in the beef broth, cheddar, tomato paste, diced pickles and cook until the cheese melts.
4.  Cover the pot and cook for 30mins on low heat.
5.  Turn off the heat and add the heavy cream and cream cheese on top and garnish with the bacon.

    *[Calories 572 | Total Fats 3.4g | Net Carbs: 3.4g | Protein 23.4g | Fiber: 0.8g]*

## Cabbage with Ground Beef Stew

[Total Time: 25 MIN| Serve: 10]

*Ingredients:*

*1 ½ lb. ground beef*

*2 lbs. green cabbage*

*½ cup unsalted butter*

*½ cup water*

*3 cups pasta sauce*

*Salt and pepper to taste*

Directions:

1. In a food processor, shred quartered cabbage.

2. In a saucepan, melt the butter and add the cabbage, water and salt and pepper to taste.

3. Cover and cook for 12-15 minutes, stirring occasionally

4. In a meanwhile, in a frying pan brown the ground beef.

5. Once browned, add the beef to the cabbage and stir well. Finally, add the pasta sauce and stir. Serve hot.

   *[Calories 307 | Total Fats 22g | Net Carbs: 12.3g | Protein 14.9g | Fiber 3.6g]*

## Slow Cooker Roast and Chicken Stew
[Total Time: 8 HR 10 MIN| Serve: 10]

*Ingredients:*

*3 lb. pot roast*

*1 lb. chicken breast  (boiled and shredded)*

*6 oz. Italian sweet sausage*

*2 cups beef broth*

*1 cup chicken stock*

*½  medium onion (chopped)*

*1 can (11 oz.) low-carb diced tomatoes*

*¼  tsp thyme*

*¼  tsp celery salt*

*1 Tbsp coconut oil*

*1 tsp basil*

*2 tsp dried dill weed*

*2 tsp garlic powder*

*2 tsp pepper*

*1 Tbsp garlic salt*

*1 tsp minced garlic*

*1 Tbsp oregano*

*1 Tbsp powdered buttermilk*

*4 tsp onion powder*

*4 tsp dried parsley*

*5 tsp red pepper flakes*

*2 tsp hot sauce*

Directions:

1. At the bottom of your Slow Cooker place roast, chicken breast, and Italian sausages. Add on the top all other ingredients and stir lightly.

2. Close the lid and cook on LOW for about 6-8 hours.

3. Once ready, flavor to taste with some additional hot sauce, salt, and pepper to your own liking and serve hot.

   *[Calories 467 | Total Fats 36g | Net Carbs: 3.7g | Protein 30g | Fiber 1.3g]*

## *Italian Fish Stew*
[Total Time: 55 MIN| Serve: 4]

*Ingredients:*

*4 Kingklip fish fillets*

*2 onions, finely chopped*

*4 garlic cloves, minced*

*2 tins peeled, chopped tomato*

*4 tbsp tomato paste*

*1 cup white wine*

*½ tsp parsley, chopped*

*¼ tsp dried oregano*

*Salt and pepper to taste*

*½ cup olive oil*

*1 cup water*

Directions:

1.	Preheat oven to 680⁰F.

2.	Sauté onion and garlic in a pot then add tinned tomatoes and tomato paste and stir.

3.	Pour the wine, parsley, oregano, salt, pepper, and water. Stir well and bring to a simmer.

4.	Let it simmer for 10-15 minutes to reduce and thicken.

5.	Meanwhile, place your fish in baking dish.

6.	When the sauce is nice and thick, pour it over fish and sprinkle with a little extra oregano.

7.	Cover the dish with foil and place in the oven to cook for 20 minutes.

8.	Take foil off and return to oven uncovered and cook for another 10 minutes.

*[Calories 315 | Total Fats 8g | Net Carbs: 12g | Protein 37g]*


## *Chicken and Mushroom Stew*
[Total Time: 45 MIN| Serve: 10]

*Ingredients:*

*8 pcs chicken thighs*

*4 tbsp butter*

*3 cloves garlic, minced*

6 cups mushrooms

1 cup chicken stock

½ tsp dried thyme

½ tsp dried oregano

½ tsp dried basil

¼ cup heavy cream

½ cup parmesan cheese, grated

1 tbsp whole-grain mustard

Directions:

1. Preheat oven to 400⁰F.

2. Season chicken thighs with salt and pepper.

3. Heat an oven-proof pan over the medium fire and melt 2 tbsp of butter.

4. Add the chicken, skin-side down, and fry both sides until golden brown, or about 2-3 minutes per side. Set aside.

5. Melt remaining 2 tbsp butter. Add garlic, thyme, oregano and basil and mushrooms, and cook, stirring occasionally. Cook until browned, about 5-6 minutes, season with salt and pepper, to taste.

6. Stir in chicken stock, then chicken back to the pan.

7. Pour everything into a baking dish with the chicken.

8. Place into oven and roast until completely cooked through for about 25-30 minutes. Set aside chicken.

9.  Transfer sauces back into the original pan.

10. Stir in heavy cream, parmesan cheese, and mustard. Bring to a boil; reduce heat and simmer until slightly reduced about 5 minutes.

11. Serve chicken immediately, topped with mushroom mixture.

*[Calories 203 | Total Fats 3g | Net Carbs: 9g | Protein 28g]*


## Beef Shin Stew

[Total Time: 3 HR 25 MIN| Serve: 8]

*Ingredients:*

*2 lb. quality shin of beef, cubed*

*4 tbsp olive oil*

*2 red onions, peeled and roughly chopped*

*3 pcs carrots, peeled and roughly chopped*

*3 sticks celery, trimmed and roughly chopped*

*4 cloves garlic, unpeeled*

*a few sprigs of fresh rosemary*

*2 bay leaves*

*2 cups mushrooms*

*2 cups baby marrows*

*Salt and pepper to taste*

*1 tbsp psyllium husk*

*2 cans tomatoes*

*⅔ Bottle red wine*

Directions:

1.  Preheat your oven to 360⁰F.

2.  In a heavy-bottomed oven-proof saucepan, heat olive oil and sauté the onions, carrots, celery, garlic, herbs, and mushrooms for 5 minutes until softened slightly.

3.  Meanwhile, roll the beef in psyllium husk.

4.  Then add meat into saucepan and stir until all ingredients are mixed.

5.  Add the tomatoes, wine and a pinch of salt and pepper and gently bring to the boil.

6.  Once boiling, turn off the heat and cover the saucepan with double thickness tinfoil and the lid.

7.  Place saucepan in the oven to cook and develop flavor for 3 hours or until the beef can be pulled apart with a spoon.

8.  Taste and add more salt if necessary.

9.  Serve and enjoy.

*[Calories 315 | Total Fats 7g | Net Carbs: 7g | Protein 20g]*

## Tuna Fish Stew

[Total Time: 25 MIN| Serve: 2]

*Ingredients:*

*1 tin tuna in water, drained*

1 tbsp butter

¼ small onion, chopped finely

1 clove garlic, minced

1tsp fresh ginger, grated

½ tin tomatoes, chopped finely

1 cup spinach, chopped finely

1 small carrot, grated

1 tsp curry powder 1 tsp turmeric

½ tsp cayenne pepper (optional)

Salt & pepper to taste

Directions:

1.  Fry onion, garlic, and ginger in butter.

2.  Add tomatoes once onions are soft.

3.  Pieces and enough water to make a stew for the spinach, carrot and tuna fish. Cook at low heat for about 15 minutes.

4.  Do not overcook spinach.

5.  Steam 2 cups of cauliflower, mash and add 1Tblsp of butter. Serve stew on top of the caulimash.

    *[Calories 253 | Total Fats 5g | Net Carbs: 7g | Protein 25g |Fiber: 2g]*

## Cauliflower 'n' Cheese Chowder
[Total Time: 30 MIN| Serve: 4]

*Ingredients:*

*4 cups cauliflower florets, chopped*

*4 bacon strips*

*1 tbsp organic butter*

*2 cloves of garlic, minced*

*1 onion, chopped fine*

*¼ cup almond flour*

*4 cups low-sodium chicken broth*

*½ cup milk*

*¼ cup light cream*

*1 cup cheddar, shredded*

*Salt and pepper to taste*

Directions:

1. Cook the bacon in a large pot. Remove from the pot when cooked and set aside.

2. Using the same pot set the heat on medium and throws in the onions. Cook for 3 minutes and then add the garlic and cauliflower florets and cook for another 5 minutes.

3. Add the flour into the pot and continuously whisk for a minute.

4. Pour the chicken broth, milk, and light cream and stir for 3 minutes.

5. Allow to simmer for 15 minutes and then turn off the heat.

6.  Add the cheddar cheese into the pot, season with salt and pepper and stir again.
7.  Serve with the chopped bacon on top.

    *[Calories 268 | Total Fats 15.9g | Net Carbs: 11.9g | Protein 19.5g | Fiber: 3.1 g]*

## *Chicken Bacon Chowder*
[Total Time: 8 HR s10 MIN| Serve: 5]

*Ingredients:*

*4 cloves garlic – minced*

*1 leek – cleaned, trimmed, and sliced*

*2 ribs celery – diced*

*1 punnet button mushrooms – sliced*

*2 medium sweet onion – thinly sliced*

*4 tbsp butter*

*2 cups chicken stock*

*6 boneless, skinless chicken breasts, butterflied*

*8 oz. cream cheese*

*1 cup heavy cream*

*1 packet streaky bacon – cooked crisp, and crumbled*

*1 tsp salt*

*1 tsp pepper*

*1 tsp garlic powder*

*1 tsp thyme*

Directions:

1.  Select low setting on your slow cooker.
2.  Place 1 cup of chicken stock, onions, garlic, mushroom, leeks, celery, 2 tbsps of butter, and the salt and pepper into your slow cooker.
3.  Put the lid on, and cook ingredients on low for 1 hour.
4.  Brown chicken breasts in a skillet with 2 tbsp of butter.
5.  Add the remaining 1 cup of chicken stock.
6.  Scrape the bottom of the skillet to remove any chicken that may have stuck to the bottom.
7.  Remove from skillet and set aside, pouring the fat from the pan over the chicken.
8.  Add in the thyme, heavy cream, garlic powder and cream cheese into your slow cooker.
9.  Stir the contents of the slow cooker until the cream cheese has melted into the dish.
10. Cut the chicken into cubes. Add the bacon and chicken cubes into the slow cooker. Stir ingredients and cook on low for 6-8 hours.

    *[Calories 355 | Total Fats 21g | Net Carbs: 6.4g | Protein 28g]*

# Vegetable Recipes

## Squash Carbonara

[Total Time: 25 MIN| Serve: 3]

*Ingredients:*

*1 pack konjac yam noodles (Shirataki)*

*2 egg yolks*

*3 tbsp squash puree*

*1/3 cup parmesan cheese, grated*

*½ cup heavy cream*

*2 tbsp organic butter*

*4 pcs pancetta*

*½ tsp dried sage*

*Salt and pepper to taste*

Directions:

1.  Boil water and soak the noodles in it for 3 minutes. Strain and set aside.

2.  Sear the pancetta on a hot pan, and chop. Reserve the fat from the pancetta

3.  Place the strained noodles on the pan cooked for the pancetta and cook for 5 minutes. Set aside.

4. On another pan (large sized) melt the butter on medium heat and allow to brown. Add the squash puree and season with sage.

5. Pour the heavy cream into the pan, add the fat from the pancetta and stir well.

6. Lastly, add the parmesan cheese into the sauceoand the mix well. Reduce the heat to low and stir until the sauce thickens.

7. Transfer the noodles into the pan with the sauce, crack the eggs and combine all the ingredients together.

*[Calories 384 | Total Fats 34.7g | Net Carbs: 2g | Protein 14g]*

## Easy Roast Tomato Sauce
[Total Time: 45 MIN| Serve: 10]

*Ingredients:*

*10 tomatoes*

*Bunch of fresh basil*

*Garlic, bulb*

*Olive oil*

*Salt and pepper*

Directions:

1. Preheat oven to 375⁰F.

2.  Slice 10 tomatoes in half lengthways

3.  Add a bunch of fresh basil.

4.  Cut an entire bulb of garlic through the middle and place each half face up in the baking dish.

5.  Immerse the tomatoes in olive oil and grind salt and pepper.

6.  Roast in the oven for about 1 hour and then turn the oven off for another 30 mins and leave to sit in the warm oven.

7.  Remove the tomatoes and allow to cool.

8.  Do not mix, as you want to squeeze the flesh and pips out of the skin and discard the skin, squeeze the garlic from the cloves and throw away the casings.

9.  Mash with a fork.

*[Calories 35 | Total Fats 1g | Net Carbs: 4g | Protein 1g | Fiber: 1]*

# Ratatouille
[Total Time: 20 MIN| Serve: 4]

*Ingredients:*

*2 large brinjals*

*1 large onion*

*2 peppers (can be green, red, and yellow)*

*2 tins of chopped tomatoes*

*1 packet baby marrows*

1 punnetmushrooms

1 packet spinach

2 ¼ cups chicken stock

Salt & pepper

2 cloves garlic  (finely chopped or pressed)

Directions:

1.   Finely chop all the ingredients.

2.   Add all the finely chopped veggies, garlic, and onion to the stock and boil on medium until the water has reduced, and the veggies have formed a thick delicious stew.

3.   Serve with 150g chunky cottage cheese, 30g cheddar or 6 tbsp Parmesan Cheese

     *[Calories 149 | Total Fats 2g | Net Carbs: 29g | Protein 7g | Fiber: 10g]*

## Cauliflower Bake
[Total Time: 40 MIN| Serve: 10]

*Ingredients:*

4 slices of bacon

2 cups broccoli

2 cups cauliflower

2 cups mushrooms

1 green pepper

*1 onion*

*1 cup cream*

*3 tbsp cheese, grated*

*2 tbsp olive oil*

Directions:

1.  Preheat oven to 360⁰F.
2.  Steam or cook the cauliflower and broccoli until tender then transfer to an oven-proof dish.
3.  Fry the bacon slices, with the mushrooms, green pepper, and onion in 2 tbsp olive oil.
4.  Pour the fried bacon and mushrooms on top of cauliflower.
5.  In a bowl, whisk 4 eggs with the cream and season to taste and pour over cauliflower or broccoli.
6.  Place in the oven to cook for 25 minutes. Take out of the oven and sprinkle with grated cheese.
7.  Place back in the oven and cook for another 5 minutes.

    *[Calories 100 | Total Fats 6g | Net Carbs: 7g| Protein 4g]*

# Caulicake

[Total Time: 55 MIN| Serve: 10]

*Ingredients:*

*1.3 lbs cauliflower florets*

*1 onion, chopped*

*3 cloves of garlic, finely chopped*

*1 tspturmeric*

*1 cup parmesan cheese, finely grated*

*1 cupmature white cheddar cheese, coarsely grated*

*8 eggs*

*1-2 tspsalt*

*2 tbsppsyllium husk*

*1 cup of cream*

*1 tbspcoconut oil*

*Sesame seeds*

*Olive oil*

Directions:

1.  Preheat oven to 360⁰F.

2.  Steam the cauliflower. Keep half of it whole and mash the rest.

3.  Sauté the onion, garlic, turmeric in the coconut oil until soft. Set aside.

4.  In a separate bowl, whisk the eggs. Add the cream, cheese, salt, and psyllium husk.

5.  Combine the cauliflower, whole and mashed with the sautéed onions and egg mixture in a bowl.

6.  Line a spring-form baking tin with greased baking paper and sprinkle with sesame seeds. Place the pan onto a baking tray.

7.  Pour in the cauliflower mix and bake in the oven for 40 minutes.

8.  As soon as it comes out of the oven, lightly prick the surface all over with a fork and drizzle with olive oil.

*[Calories 160 | Total Fats 11g | Net Carbs: 5g | Protein 8g]*

## Spiced Kale "Meatballs"

[Total Time: 25 MIN| Serve: 8]

*Ingredients:*

*4 Tbsp olive oil*

*1 cup almond flour*

*1 bunch of kale leaves*

*1 green chili, chopped*

*¼ tsp red chili powder*

*¼ tsp turmeric powder*

*1 tsp cumin seed powder*

*¼ tsp ginger, minced*

*Black salt or salt as per taste*

*1 tsp cooking soda or baking soda (optional)*

*Water for batter*

Directions:

1. In a bowl, mix all the ingredients together.
2. Combine and knead the batter with your finger. The consistency should be not too thick nor too thin. Make a kale "meatballs".
3. Heat oil in a frying pan. Place a kale "meatballs" in the hot oil one by one.
4. Fry few at a time don't cluster with too many. When they get golden color from one side, turn and cook on another side.
5. Remove the fries with slotted spoon and place over absorbent napkins.
6. Serve hot.

    *[Calories 125 | Total Fats 6.2g | Net Carbs: 13g | Protein 6g | Fiber 4.8g]*

## *Pumpkin Carbonara*
[Total Time: 30 MIN| Serve: 4]

*Ingredients:*

*5 oz Pancetta*

*¼ cup Heavy cream*

2 tbsp Butter

½ tsp Sage, dried

Black pepper

1 packet Shirataki noodles

2 Egg yolks

1/3 cup Parmesan cheese

3 tbsp Pumpkin puree

Salt


Directions:

1.   Boil a pot of water and add noodles, cook for 3 minutes then drain. Dry completely and put aside until needed.

2.   Chop pancetta, heat skillet and cook pancetta until crispy. Reserve oil and put pancetta aside until needed.

3.   Heat a small pot and add butter, cook, until it gets brown then add pureeoand sage.

4.   Add pancetta, fat and cream, mix together until thoroughly combined.

5.   Heat pan that had in fat on a high flame and stirs fry noodles for 5 minutes.

6.   Add cheese to pumpkin mixture, combine and lower heat; cook until sauce gets thick.

7. Add pancetta and noodles to sauce, tossothen add yolks and mix together; cook for 3ominutes.

8. Serve.

   *[Calories 384 | Total Fats 34.7g | Net Carbs: 2g | Protein 14g | Fiber: 2g]*


## One Pot Italian Sausage Meal

[Total Time: 25 MIN| Serve: 2]

*Ingredients:*

*1 Tbsp Onion*

*¼ Cup Parmesan cheese*

*½ Tsp Oregano*

*¼ Tsp Salt*

*3 Sausage links*

*4 oz. Mushrooms*

*¼ Cup Mozzarella cheese (shredded)*

*½ Tsp Basil*

*¼ Tsp Red pepper flakes*


Directions:

1. Set oven to 350⁰F.

2. Heat a cast iron skillet until it starts to smoke then add sausages and cook until almost done.

3. Slice onion and mushrooms and remove sausages from the pot and add sliced veggies and cook for 3 minutes until golden.

4. Slice sausages and add to skillet along with seasonings. Add parmesan and stir to combine.

5. Place skillet into the oven and cook for 10 minutes then top with mozzarella and cook until cheese melts.

6. Serve.

*[Calories 500 | Total Fats 38g | Net Carbs: 4.5g | Protein 30g | Fiber: 2g]*

# No-Sweat Spinach Salad

[Total Time: 15 MIN| Serve: 4]

*Ingredients:*

*4 cups baby spinach*

*4 strips of bacon, cooked and crumbled*

*4 tbsp blue cheese, crumbled*

*¼ cup macadamia nuts, chopped*

*½ onion, sliced thin*

*¼ cup vinaigrette*

Directions:

1. Clean the baby spinach thoroughly and dry.

2. Place in a salad bowl.

3. Sprinkle the blue cheese, bacon, and nuts on top.

4. Add the onions and then drizzle with vinaigrette.

   *[Calories 690 | Total Fats 66.9g | Net Carbs: 16.5g | Protein 13.9g | Fiber 6.7g]*


## Baked Cheesy Zucchini

[Total Time: 40 MIN| Serve: 2]

*Ingredients:*

*2 pcs zucchini, peeled and grated*

*¼ cup parmesan cheese, grated*

*½ cup mozzarella cheese, grated*

*1 clove of garlic*

*2 organic eggs*

*3 tbsp organic butter, (separate 1 tbsp)*

*1 tsp salt*


Directions:

1. Place the grated zucchini in a bowl and season with salt. Let it rest for 25 minutes.

2. Set oven to 400⁰F.

3. After the zucchini has rested for 25 minutes place it in the middle of a dishtowel and squeeze out the liquid from it. Set aside.

4. Heat the 2 tbsp of butter in a pan and sauté the garlic for about a minute. Add the parmesan cheese

and then throw in the zucchini to the pan and cook for 6 minutes. Stir occasionally.

5. Transfer into an oven-safe dish and then sprinkle with the grated mozzarella.

6. Bake in the oven for 10 minutes or until the cheese has melted.

7. While waiting for the zucchini to bake, fry the eggs using the remaining 1 tbsp of butter.

8. Remove the zucchini from the oven when done baking and serve topped with the butter-fried egg.

*[Calories 552 | Total Fats 42g | Net Carbs: 10g | Protein 37g]*

## Level-Up Spinach Salad

[Total Time: 25 MIN| Serve: 2]

*Ingredients:*

*2 tbsp organic butter*

*1 small onion, sliced thin*

*3 cups baby spinach*

*2 organic eggs, cooked hard boiled*

*2 bacon strips, cooked and chopped*

*4 tbsp slivered almonds*

*4 tbsp gorgonzola cheese*

*For the dressing*

*2 tbsp extra virgin olive oil*

*2 tbsp balsamic vinegar*

*Salt and pepper to taste*

Directions:

1. Heat the butter in a pan over medium fire.

2. Add the onions, season with salt and pepper and cook for 15 minutes, or until the onions caramelize.

3. While waiting for the onions to cook, prepare the dressing by whisking all the ingredients in a bowl. Set aside.

4. Also prepare the salad by adding the spinach to the bowl and then top with the sliced hard-boiled eggs, cheese, almonds, caramelized onion, and bacon.

5. Drizzle with the dressing and toss to incorporate all the ingredients.

   *[Calories 607 | Total Fats 52g | Net Carbs: 13g | Protein 20g | Fiber: 2.6g]*

## *Pizza in Mushroom Cups*

[Total Time: 20 MIN| Serve: 3]

*Ingredients:*

*3 large Portobello mushroom caps*

*3 tsp pizza seasoning*

*3 tomato, slices*

*½ cup fresh basil leaves, chopped*

*12 slices pepperoni*

¼ cup mozzarella cheese

¼ cup cheddar cheese

¼ cup Monterey Jack

½ tbsp olive oil

## Directions:

1. Set the oven at 450⁰F.

2. Place the mushroom caps on a baking sheet lined with parchment paper and drizzle with olive oil.

3. Season with the pizza seasoning and top with the basil, tomato slices, cheeses, and season again.

4. Place in the oven to bake for 5-6 minutes or until the cheese has melted.

5. Get the baking sheet out of the oven and then top with the pepperoni and place back in the oven and bake until the pepperoni is cooked.

   *[Calories 276| Total Fats 21g | Net Carbs: 6g | Protein 19g | Fiber: 2 g]*


## *Spinach Cheese 'n' Bacon Log*

[Total Time: 1 HR 15 MIN| Serve: 5]

*Ingredients:*

*2 ½ cups cheddar cheese, shredded*

*2 tbsp chipotle seasoning*

*30 bacon slices*

*2 tsp Mrs. Dash seasoning*

*5 cups spinach*

Directions:

1.  Set oven to 375⁰F.
2.  Place bacon in a weaving pattern on a baking sheet lined with foil and season with spices.
3.  Top bacon with cheese leaving a 1-inch space all around the edge. Add spinach and push it down and roll the bacon together into a log.
4.  Sprinkle with salt and place into oven for 60 minutes.
5.  Cool for 15 minutes and slice.
6.  Serve.

    *[Calories 432 | Total Fats 38.2g | Net Carbs: 3g | Protein 32.8g | Fiber 3 g]*

## Hearty Salad

[Total Time: 10 MIN| Serve: 2]

*Ingredients:*

*1 Hard Boiled Egg grated*

*2 slices of country ham, finely sliced*

*1.05 oz cheddar cheese*

*1 tomato finely diced*

*2 tbsp mayo*

*1 cup finely sliced crispy lettuce*

2 spring onions finely chopped

½ green peppers finely chopped

Directions:

1.  Combine all the ingredients and then add the mayo

    *[Calories 214 | Total Fats 14.6g | Net Carbs: 9.5g | Protein 12.2g]*


## Spinach and Goat Cheese Salad
[Total Time: 20 MIN| Serve: 2]

*Ingredients:*

*4 Cups Spinach*

*4 Strawberries*

*1 ½ Cups Goat cheese (grated)*

*½ Cup Almond flakes (toasted)*

*4 Tbsp Vinaigrette*

Directions:

1.  Set oven to 400⁰F and use parchment paper to line a baking sheet. Cut paper in half.

2.  Grate cheese onto sheet and form into circles.

3.  Bake for 10 minutes until golden. Gently lift parchment paper and shape cheese around bowls, cool and remove.

4.  Toss spinach with vinaigrette and place into a hardened bowl. Top with almonds and strawberries.

6.  Serve.

*[Calories 645 | Total Fats 54.2g | Net Carbs: 9.8g | Protein 33.2g | Fiber 4g]*

## Greek Eggplant Salad

[Total Time: 1 HR 10 MIN| Serve: 6]

*Ingredients:*

*2 lbs. Eggplants*

*4 Garlic cloves, crushed*

*Parsley, chopped*

*½ Tsp Salt*

*2.6 oz. Onion, chopped*

*Lemon juice*

*¼ Cup extra virgin Olive oil*

Directions:

1. Set oven to 350⁰F and rinse eggplants and pat dry then place on a baking sheet.

2. Bake for 60 minutes until soft.

3. Add onion to food processor and pulse until fine. Add oil to a bowl and transfer onion to a clean cloth or fine sieve and squeeze onion juice into the oil. Discard onion solids or save for future use.

4. Add garlic, parsley and lemon juice to bowl also and whisk together.

5.  When eggplants are cooled, slice and scoop insides into a bowl and mash. Add oil mixture to eggplants and stir. Add pepper and salt to taste.

6.  Serve.

*[Calories 130 | Total Fats 9.4g | Net Carbs: 12g | Protein 33.2g | Fiber: 4g]*

## Egg and Avocado Salad

[Total Time: 15 MIN| Serve: 2]

*Ingredients:*

*1 Avocado, sliced*

*½ Cup Yogurt (full fat)*

*2 Tsp Dijon mustard*

*4 Eggs*

*4 Cups Mixed greens*

*2 Garlic cloves (smashed)*

*Salt*

*Black pepper*

*Fresh herbs*

Directions:

1.  Cook eggs until hard-boiled and then place into a pan with cold water.

2.  Prepare the dressing by mixing yogurt, mustard, and garlic together. Season with black pepper and salt.

3.  Rinse and drain green and place into a bowl.

4. Top with sliced avocados and slice eggs into quarters and top salad; drizzle with dressing with a dash of pepper and salt.

5. Serve.

   *[Calories 436 | Total Fats 36.3g | Net Carbs: 13.7g | Protein 17g | Fiber: 7.6g]*

## Tricolor Salad

[Total Time: 10 MIN| Serve: 2]

*Ingredients:*

*1 Avocado*

*4.5 oz. Mozzarella cheese*

*8 Kalamata Olives*

*2 Tbsp Pesto*

*Salt*

*Black pepper*

*4 Tomatoes*

*2 Tbsp Olive oil (extra virgin)*

*Basil (chopped)*

Directions:

1. Slice tomatoes and avocados. Remove seeds from olives and slice.

2. Add all sliced ingredients to a bowl and top with cheese, oil, and pesto.

3. Add pepper and salt to taste.

4. Serve.

*[Calories 581 | Total Fats 50.7g | Net Carbs: 17.6g | Protein 19.2g | Fiber: 9g]*

# Cucumber Strawberry Salsa and Grilled Halloumi
[Total Time: 20 MIN| Serve: 4]

*Ingredients:*

*14.1 oz. Halloumi cheese*

*5.3 oz. Cucumber*

*Lime juice (freshly squeezed from 1 lime)*

*1 Tbsp mint (chopped)*

*2 Tbsp Olive oil (extra-virgin)*

*1 Tbsp Butter*

*Black pepper*

*1 Cup Strawberries*

*1 Jalapeno*

*1 Garlic clove*

*2 Tbsp Basil (chopped)*

*1 Tbsp Balsamic vinegar*

*¼ Tsp Salt*

## Directions:

1. Chop strawberries, peel cucumber and dice; remove seeds from pepper and chop.

2.   Chop herbs and crush garlic and add to a bowl. Add lime juice, vinegar, and oil and whisk together.

3.   Add dressing to chopped vegetables and fruits, toss and add pepper and salt to taste.

4.   Slice cheese, heat butter in a skillet and cook for 3 minutes until golden per side.

5.   Top grilled cheese with salsa and serve.

*[Calories 449 | Total Fats 37.7g | Net Carbs: 8.1g | Protein 20.8g | Fiber: 1.3 g]*

## Green Veggie Salad

[Total Time: 10 MIN| Serve: 6]

*Ingredients:*

*1 cup green beans, steamed lightly*

*1 cup broccoli florets, steamed lightly*

*1 small tomato, finely sliced*

*1 cup lettuce*

*1 round feta*

*¼ cup toasted sunflower seeds, roasted*

*1 hard-boiled egg, chopped*

*For dressing:*

*1 tbsp olive oil*

*Salt and pepper to taste*

*½ lemon juice*

Directions:

1.  Place all the vegetables in a salad bowl.
2.  Crumble the feta and sprinkle it along with the roasted pumpkin seeds and egg on top of the salad.
3.  In a small bowl, pour the olive oil, add lemon juice, then add salt and pepper, and whisk together. Drizzle this dressing on top of the salad.
4.  Toss gently before serving.

*[Calories 45 | Total Fats 3g | Net Carbs: 3g | Protein 1g]*

## Bacon, Lettuce, Tomato Salad
[Total Time: 15 MIN| Serve: 4]

*Ingredients:*

*1 cup of lettuce*

*1 spring onion*

*1 tomato*

*¼ cup toasted pumpkin seeds*

*Grated boiled egg*

*Sliced avocado*

*4 rashers of crispy bacon (crumbled)*

*For dressing:*

*1 tbsp apple cider vinegar*

*1 tsp lemon juice*

*½ a finely crushed clove of garlic*

*1 tbsp olive oil and some finely crushed fresh ginger (optional)*

Directions:

1.  In a large bowl combine salad ingredient.
    This can all be done at home and taken to work.
2.  For dressing: In a separate container mix dressing ingredient.
3.  Allow the dressing to sit for a few hours.
4.  Pour the dressing over the salad when you are ready to eat.

    *[Calories 288 | Total Fats 26g | Net Carbs: 7.4g | Protein 9.9g]*

## Broccoli Salad

[Total Time: 10 MIN| Serve: 4]

*Ingredients:*

*1 cup broccoli*

*2 medium celery stalks*

*½ cup mushroom pieces (fried)*

*¼ cup Cherry tomatoes*

*1 tbsp olive oil*

*2 cups Lettuce*

*1 tbsp balsamic vinegar*

*½ cup pumpkin seeds roasted dry in a pan*

Directions:

1.  Place all ingredients into a bowl, mix and enjoy.

    *[Calories 143 | Total Fats 11.6g | Net Carbs: 6.8g | Protein 5.5g | Fiber: 2g]*

## Bacon with Cheesy Cauliflower Mash
[Total Time: 30 MIN| Serve: 3]

*Ingredients:*

*4 cups cauliflower florets, chopped*

*3 tbsp heavy cream*

*¼ tsp garlic powder*

*Salt and pepper to taste*

*4 bacon strips, cooked and chopped*

*1 cup cheddar cheese, shredded*

Directions:

1. In an oven-safe bowl, mix the chopped cauliflower florets, heavy cream, butter, and season with the garlic powder, salt, and pepper.

2. Place the bowl in the microwave and cook on high for 20 minutes or until the cauliflower is soft.

3. Pour the cooked cauliflower into a food processor and add the bacon and cheddar cheese.

4. Pulse until you achieve a smooth consistency.

5. Serve with a dab on of butter on top.

   *[Calories 590| Total Fats 51g | Net Carbs: 6g | Protein 22g | Fiber 5.0g]*

## *Crispy Baked Tofu and Bok Choy Salad*

[Total Time: 45 MIN| Serve: 3]

*Ingredients:*

*For Tofu:*

*1 tbsp soy sauce*

*1 tbsp water*

*1 tbsp rice wine vinegar*

*15 oz extra firm tofu*

*1 tbsp sesame oil*

*2 tsp garlic*

*½ lemon juice*

*For Salad:*

*1 green onion*

*3 tbsp coconut oil*

*1 tbsp sambal oelek*

*½ lime juice*

*9 oz Bok Choy*

*2 tbsp Cilantro, chopped*

*2 tbsp soy sauce*

*1 tbsp peanut butter*

*7 drops stevia liquid*

## Directions:

1. Wrap tofu in a clean cloth and press for 6 hours until dry.

2. Combine soy sauce, water, vinegar, lemon juice, sesame oil and garlic in a bowl and cube tofu. Add to marinade, cover with plastic and put aside for 30 minutes or overnight if possible.

3. Set oven to 350⁰F. Uses parchment paper to line a baking sheet and place marinated tofu on the sheet. Bake for 35 minutes.

4. Prepare to dress for salad by combining all ingredients except bok choy. Chop book choy finely and toss in dressing.

5. Top bok choy with baked tofu and serve.

   *[Calories 442 | Total Fats 35g | Net Carbs: 5.7g | Protein 25g | Fiber 1.7g]*

## Creamed Spinach

[Total Time: 15 MIN| Serve: 1]

*Ingredients:*

*2 cup spinach*

*½ small onion, chopped*

*¼ cups water*

*½ stock cube*

*1 clove of garlic, chopped*

*¼ cups heavy cream*

*2 tbsp butter*

*Salt and pepper to taste*

Directions:

1.  Place spinach and onion to a pan with water and heat over the medium-high fire.
2.  Add the stock cube and garlic and allow to steam for 8-10 minutes or until all the water has evaporated and the spinach is very soft.
3.  Pour in the heavy cream and butter and then season with salt and pepper. Cooking until it thickens.
4.  Using a hand-held blender blitz the spinach until fairly smooth.
5.  Serve while hot

*[Calories 200 | Total Fats 23g | Net Carbs: 3g | Protein 7g]*

## Cheesy Zoodles with Fresh Basil
[Total Time: 15 MIN| Serve: 3]

*Ingredients:*

*2 cups zucchini noodles (zoodles)*

*2 Tbsp fresh chopped basil*

*¼ cup pecorino Romano cheese, shaved*

*¼ cup Grana Padano cheese, grated*

*3 Tbsp salted butter*

*3 cloves mashed garlic*

*1 tsp red pepper flakes*

1 Tbsp chopped red pepper

1 Tbsp coconut oil

Salt and fresh cracked pepper to taste

Directions:

1.  In a frying pan over medium heat, melt butter and coconut oil. Add in garlic, chopped red pepper, and red pepper flakes. Sauté for 1 minute only.

2.  Add in the zoodles and let cook for 1-2 minutes. Turn off heat and toss with fresh basil. Toss lightly.

3.  Add in Pecorino Romano cheese and toss.

4.  Finally, sprinkle on top with grated Grana Padano cheese.

5.  Serve immediately.

    *[Calories 314 | Total Fats 26g | Net Carbs: 6.1g | Protein 15g | Fiber 2.3g]*

## *Veggie Burger Patties*
[Total Time: 20 MIN| Serve: 4]

*Ingredients:*

*2 cups Brussels sprouts*

*3 organic eggs*

*1 cup parmesan cheese, grated*

*1 ½ goat cheese*

*½ cup green onion, chopped*

*1/3 cup almond flour*

1 cup parmesan cheese

1 ½ goat cheese

Salt and pepper to taste

Directions:

1. Thoroughly wash the Brussels sprouts and place in the food processor to shred into pieces.

2. Transfer the Brussels sprouts to a bowl and add the parmesan cheese and almond flour into the bowl. Season with salt and pepper.

3. In another bowl, whisk the eggs and then pour over the Brussels sprouts mixture. Combine well using your hands.

4. Create burger patties, about 4 oz. each and then fry in a greased cast iron skillet for about 2 minutes on each side, or until crispy.

   [Calories 182 | Total Fats 11g | Net Carbs: 7g | Protein 14g | Fiber 3g]

## Mascarpone Zucchini Rolls
[Total Time: 15 MIN| Serve: 2]

Ingredients:

1 large zucchini cut thin using a mandolin

6 oz. mascarpone cheese

1 tsp dill, dried

1 tsp mint, dried

*Salt and pepper to taste*

*1 tbsp melted butter*

Directions:

1. Brush the zucchini slices with the melted butter and season with salt and pepper

2. Heat your grill and place the zucchini. Cook for 2 minutes on each side.

3. In a bowl, combine the mascarpone, dill, and mint and whisk well.

4. Equally, scoop the mascarpone mixture on top of the grilled zucchini and spread.

5. Roll the zucchini and secure with toothpicks. Serve and consume immediately.

   *[Calories 186| Total Fats 14g | Net Carbs: 3g | Protein 13g | Fiber: 1 g]*


## Tasty Cauliflower Rice
[Total Time: 25 MIN| Serve: 2]

*Ingredients:*

*4 cups cauliflower florets*

*1 small onion, diced*

*2 cloves of garlic, minced*

*1 ½ tsp garlic powder*

*1½ tsp cumin*

*1 ½ tsp chili powder*

*Salt to taste*

*1 tbsp ghee*

*1 cup cheddar cheese, shredded*

*4 tbsp sour cream*

Directions:

1.  Heat the ghee in a skillet over medium fire.
2.  Add the onions into the hot pan and sauté for 3 minutes.
3.  While waiting for the onions to cook place the cauliflower florets in a food processor and pulse until they are chopped.
4.  Throw in the garlic into the pan and sauté for another half a minute.
5.  Add the chopped cauliflower to the pan, along with the garlic powder, cumin, chili powder, and season with salt.
6.  Cook the cauliflower for 12-15 minutes or until tender.
7.  Turn off the heat and transfer the cauliflower rice into serving bowls.
8.  Top with the shredded cheese and sour cream while hot.

*[Calories 618| Total Fats 48g | Net Carbs: 17g | Protein 27g | Fiber: 27g]*

## Roquefort Spinach, Zoodles and Bacon Salad

[Total Time: 5 MIN| Serve: 5]

*Ingredients:*

*4 cups of zucchini noodles*

*1 cup fresh broccoli*

*½ cup crumbled bacon*

*1 cup fresh spinach*

*1/3 cup Roquefort, bleu cheese, crumbled*

*1/3 cup bleu cheese dressing*

*Fresh cracked pepper (to taste)*

Directions:

1.  In a deep bowl add all the ingredients together and toss lightly with a wooden spoon.

2.  Serve and enjoy.

    *[Calories 81.2 | Total Fats 3.1g | Net Carbs: 9.5g | Protein 6g | Fiber: 3.05g]*

## Spinach and Cheese Stuffed Mushrooms

[Total Time: 20 MIN| Serve: 6]

*Ingredients:*

*12 large mushroom caps with stems*

*1 cream cheese*

*1 cup cooked, chopped spinach*

*1 Tbsp garlic, minced*

*1 tsp red pepper flakes*

*2 scallions, finely chopped*

*1 tsp salt*

*1 tsp fresh cracked pepper*

*3 tsp extra virgin olive oil*

*2 Tbsp almond, ground*

*2 Tbsp Parmesan cheese*

*1 tsp granulated garlic*

*1 Tbsp fresh flat leaf parsley, finely chopped*

Directions:

1. Preheat oven to 400⁰F.

2. First, remove the mushrooms stems and chop the stems into small pieces.

3. Heat 2 tbsp of olive a frying pan and sauté mushroom stems for about 5 minutes.

4. In a small bowl mix cooked mushroom stems, cream cheese, chopped spinach, scallions, minced garlic, red pepper flakes, salt, and pepper.

5. Then mix parmesan cheese, ground almonds, granulated garlic and parsley in another small bowl.

6. Fill the inside of the mushroom tops with the mushroom mixture and cheese. Then add the ground almonds mixture over the top of each mushroom.

7. Sprinkle the last tsp of oil over the mushroom caps and add a little extra cheese on the top.

8.   Bake in oven about 12 minutes.

9.   Serve hot.

   *[Calories 138.32 | Total Fats 6.36g | Net Carbs: 6.98g | Protein 11.75g | Fiber 5.24g]*


## Baked Broccoli with Mushrooms and Parmesan
[Total Time: 35 MIN| Serve: 2]

*Ingredients:*

*4 cups broccoli*

*2 cups mushrooms (chopped fine)*

*2 Tbsp minced garlic*

*½ tsp dried regano*

*3 Tbsp grated Parmesan*

*Salt and ground black pepper to taste*

Directions:

1.   Preheat oven to 300⁰F. Line a baking sheet with parchment paper.

2.   Wash and slice broccoli into florets.

3.   In a bowl, toss broccoli and finely chopped mushrooms in olive oil.

4.   Season with dried oregano, salt, and pepper to taste.

5.   Spread all vegetables evenly over the prepared baking pan.

6.   Bake for 20-25 minutes until the broccoli is browned.

7. When done, leave to cool 5 minutes, sprinkle with Parmesan cheese serve.

*[Calories 138.26 | Total Fats 3.51g | Net Carbs: 4.86g | Protein 12.16g | Fiber 3.33g]*

## Ail Creamy Brussels sprouts

[Total Time: 15 MIN| Serve: 1]

*Ingredients:*

*10 Brussels sprouts*

*4 cloves garlic*

*¼ cup cream cheese*

*2 Tbsp extra virgin olive oil*

*1 tsp Balsamic vinegar*

*Salt and pepper to taste*

Directions:

1. Clean the Brussels sprouts discarding the first leaves and cut into julienne strips.
2. Peel and chop the garlic cloves.
3. In a frying pan, heat the olive oil and saute the Brussels Sprouts and garlic,
4. When the garlic and sprouts areotender, turn off the heat andoadd the cheese. Letosit for a couple of minutes.
5. Transfer tooplate and serve.

*[Calories 223.26 | Total Fats 12.55g | Net Carbs: 5.21g | Protein 9.27g | Fiber: 6.22g]*

## Spicy Cauliflower with Sujuk Sausages

[Total Time: 30 MIN| Serve: 4]

*Ingredients:*

*4 cups frozen cauliflower*

*8 oz sujuk sausages sliced (or red pastrami)*

*1 green pepper, chopped*

*1 tsp Cajun seasoning*

*½ onion, chopped*

*2 tbsp minced garlic*

*2 tbsp olive oil*

Directions:

1. In a frying pan, sauté onion in olive oil for 2-3 minutes.

2. Squeeze the liquid from chopped cauliflower and add it to the pan. Sauté the cauliflower with onion 5-10 minutes.

3. Add in Cajun seasoning and mix. Add in chopped sujuk sausages or pastrami and green peppers.

4. Toss and cook until about 5 minutes. Transfer to the plates. Serve.

*[Calories 181 | Total Fats 10g | Net Carbs: 9g | Protein 14g]*

## Electric Pressure Cooker Bok Choy Salad

[Total Time: 10 MIN| Serve: 3]

*Ingredients:*

*1 bunch Bok choy, trimmed*

*1 cup or more water*

*Salt*

*Olive oil*

*Lime*

Directions:

1. Place the stems in your Electric pressure cooker and pour one cup or more water to just cover the stems.

2. Close and lock the lid of the pressure cooker. Turn the heat up to high and when the cooker reaches pressure, lower to the heat to the minimum required by the cooker to maintain pressure.

3. Cook for 5-7 minutes at high pressure.

4. When time is up, open the cooker by Slowly releasing the pressure.

5. Pull out the leaves and stems with tongs, and put on a small serving plate.

6. Dress with salt and olive oil before serving. Sprinkle some lime juice.

*[Calories 36.4 | Total Fats 0.56g | Net Carbs: 3.1g | Protein 4.2g | Fiber 2.8g]*

## Desserts & Sweet Fat Bombs

### All-stars Peanut-Butter Cookies

[Total Time: 1 HR 15 MIN| Serve: 18]

*Ingredients:*

*2 cups peanut butter*

*¼ cup Erythritol*

*2 eggs*

*1 ¼ cups coconut flour*

*2 tsp baking soda*

*2 tsp peanut extract*

*½ tsp kosher salt*

Directions:

1. Preheat oven to 345⁰F.

2. In a bowl beat the peanut butter, coconut flour and Erythritol with an electric mixer (MEDIUM speed) until fluffy. Reduce speed to LOW and add in the eggs, baking soda, vanilla, and salt.

3. With your handsomake balls from the batter and place on parchment-lined baking pan. Bake 10 to 15 minutes. When ready, cool slightly and then move from the stove to coolocompletely. Ready. Serve.

*[Calories 182.5 | Total Fats 14.67g | Net Carbs: 8.65g | Protein 7g | Fiber 1.96g]*

## Almond Chocolate Brownies

[Total Time: 35 MIN| Serve: 16]

*Ingredients:*

*3 eggs*

*4 oz dark chocolate, unsweetened*

*1/2 cup coconut oil*

*1 cup almond flour*

*1 cup walnuts, chopped*

*2 Tbsp cocoa, unsweetened*

*1 tsp vanilla essence*

*2 cups granulated sweetener Stevia or Erythritol*

*1 tsp baking soda*

*Pinch of salt*

Directions:

1.  Preheat the oven to 350⁰F.

2.  In a container, add almond flour, sweetener, cocoa, salt and baking soda. With an electric mixer, blend the ingredients on the lowest setting until combined well.

3.  Melt the chocolate and the coconut oil together. Stir thoroughly.

4.  Add eggs and vanilla essence to the flour and mix on a medium speed until a thick batter is formed.

5.  Add the butter/chocolate mix to the batter continuing on medium speed until an even texture is formed.

6.  Line a slice tin or square baking tin with wax paper.

7.  Fold in chopped walnut then turn the batter into your

8.  slice tin.

9.  Bake for 25 minutes.

10. Cut into 16 Brownies and serve.

*[Calories 207.88 | Total Fats 20.72g | Net Carbs: 5.38g | Protein 5.14g | Fiber 2.82g]*

## Almond Chocolate Cookies
[Total Time: 25 MIN| Serve: 12]

*Ingredients:*

*2 cups almond meal*

*1 ½ tsp almond extract*

*4 Tbsp cocoa powder*

*5 Tbsp coconut oil, melted*

*2 Tbsp almond milk*

*4 Tbsp agave nectar*

*2 tsp vanilla extract*

*1/8 tsp baking soda*

*1/8 tsp salt*

Directions:

1. Preheat oven to 340⁰F degrees.

2. In a deep bowl mix salt, cocoa powder, almond meal and baking soda.

3. In a separate bowl, whisk together melted coconut oil, almond milk, almond and vanilla extract and maple syrup. Merge the almond meal mixture with almond milk mixture and mix well.

4. In a greased baking pan pour the batter evenly. Bake for 10-15 minutes.

5. Once ready let cool on a wire rack and serve.
   *[Calories 79.32 | Total Fats 5.94g | Net Carbs: 7.2g | Protein 0.46g | Fiber 0.61g]*

## *Carrot Flowers Muffins*
[Total Time: 50 MIN| Serve: 12]

*Ingredients:*

*2 eggs*

*2 cups shredded carrots*

*¼ cup coconut flour*

*½ cup coconut oil*

*1 tsp vanilla extract*

*¼ cup Erythritol*

*2 tsp ground cinnamon*

*1 tsp baking powder*

Directions:

1.  Preheat oven to 350⁰F. Prepare 12 muffin tins.

2.  In your food processor, add in carrots, eggs, coconut oil, Erythritol, and vanilla. Blend together until combined.

3.  In a separate bowl, mix together coconut flour, cinnamon, and baking powder.

4.  Pour the carrot mixture into the dry ingredients and mix until completely combined.

5.  Pour carrot mixture into the muffin tin and bake for about 30-35 minutes.

6.  Remove from the oven, and let cool for at least 30 minutes. Serve.

    *[Calories 127.55 | Total Fats 10.4g | Net Carbs: 8.81g | Protein 1.53g | Fiber 0.91g]*


## Coconut Jelly Cake

[Total Time: 30 MIN| Serve: 18]

*Ingredients:*

*1 cup coconut flour*

*½ cup butter, softened*

*2 tbsp raspberry jelly*

*½ cup coconut sugar*

*3 cups desiccated coconut*

*1 egg*

*2/3 cup coconut milk*

*1 cup boiling water*

*1 cup cold water*

*½ cup double thick cream*

Directions:

1.  Preheat oven to 360⁰F. Grease a patty pan.

2.  In a bowl beat coconut sugar and butter until light.

3.  Add in egg and beat until well combined. Gently fold in half the coconut flour and half the milk. Repeat with remaining flour and milk.

4.  Spoon mixture into patty pan. Bake for 15 to 20 minutes. Once ready, let cool cakes on a wire rack.

5.  Stir boiling water and jelly together in a bowl until dissolved.

6.  Stir in cold water and place in refrigerator for 1 hour.

7.  Place coconut into a large bowl.

8.  Cut each cake into the half.

9.  Stick halves back together using 1 tsp of cream.

10. Using a spoon lower cakes, 1 cake at a time, into jelly.

11. Toss cakes in coconut.

12. When ready, place onto a lined tray and refrigerate for 1 hour.

*[Calories 146.51 | Total Fats 14.31g | Net Carbs: 4.21g | Protein 1.83g | Fiber: 2.16g]*

## Cottage Pumpkin Pie Ice Cream

[Total Time: 15 MIN| Serve: 6]

*Ingredients:*

*½ cup toasted pecans, chopped*

*3 egg yolks*

*2 Tbsp butter, salted*

*2 cups coconut milk*

*½ cup pumpkin puree*

*1 tsp pumpkin spice*

*½ cup cottage cheese*

*½ tsp chia seeds*

*1/3 cup Erythritol*

*20 drops liquid Nutria*

Directions:

1. Place all ingredients into a container of your immersion blender. Blend all of the ingredients together into a smooth mixture.

2. Add mixture to your ice cream machine.

3. Churn the ice cream using ice cream maker manufacturer's instructions.

4. Serve in a chilled and enjoy.

[*Calories 233.69 | Total Fats 21.74g | Net Carbs: 6.87g | Protein 5.49g | Fiber: 1.95g*]

## Divine Keto Chocolate Biscotti

[Total Time: 25 MIN| Serve: 8]

*Ingredients:*

*1 egg*

*2 cups whole almonds*

*2 Tbsp flax seeds*

*1 cup shredded coconut, unsweetened*

*1 cup coconut oil*

*1 cup cacao powder*

*1/4 cup Xylitol or Stevia sweetener*

*1 tsp salt*

*1 tsp baking soda*

Directions:

1. Preheat oven to 350⁰F.

2. In a food processor blend the almonds with the flax seeds.

3. Add in the rest of ingredients and mix well.

4. Place the dough on a piece of aluminum foil to shape into eight biscotti-shaped slices.

5. Bake in preheated oven for 12 minutes.

6. Let cool and serve.

*[Calories 276.56 | Total Fats 25.44g | Net Carbs: 9.19g | Protein 8.24g | Fiber: 5.2g]*

## Halloween Pumpkin Ice Cream

[Total Time: 15 MIN| Serve: 6]

*Ingredients:*

*1 cup almond milk (unsweetened)*

*1 cup coconut milk*

*1 cup pumpkin puree*

*2 ½ tsp ground cinnamon*

*1 tsp pure vanilla extract*

*½ tsp ground ginger*

*½ tsp nutmeg*

*1/8 tsp sea salt*

*Thickener:*

*½ tsp guar gum or 1 tbsp gelatin dissolved in 1/4 cup boiling water*

Directions:

1. Put the coconut milk in a blender and purée until smooth.

2. Pour into the ice cream machine or blender and churn well. Serve in chilled glasses.

3. Freeze for about an hour or refrigerate until cold.

5.  Add the almond milk, pumpkin puree, vanilla, cinnamon, ginger, nutmeg, and salt, plus a thickener. Purée until smooth.
6.  Serve.

    *[Calories 118.25 | Total Fats 11.3g | Net Carbs: 4.73g | Protein 1.35g | Fiber: 1.4g]*

## Hemp and Chia Seeds Cream

[Total Time: 20 MIN| Serve: 3]

*Ingredients:*

*1 ¼ cup coconut milk*

*2 Tbsp hemp powder*

*2 sheets of unflavored gelatin*

*3 Tbsp chia seeds*

Directions:

1.  In a saucepan over low heat add the coconut milk and dissolve the lucuma powder.
2.  Cut the gelatin into pieces and add it to the milk. Stir until dissolved completely.
3.  Add chia seeds and stir occasionally until mixture thickens about 15 minutes. Pour the mixture into individual containers and allow cool before putting them in the refrigerator for at least 2 hours before serving. Enjoy!

*[Calories 202.43 | Total Fats 160.45g | Net Carbs: 8.12g | Protein 2.59g |Fiber: 3.14g]*

## Homemade Nut Bars

[Total Time: 15 MIN| Serve: 10]

*Ingredients:*

*1 cup almonds*

*½ cup hazelnuts, chopped*

*1 cup peanuts*

*1 cup shredded coconut*

*1 cup almond butter*

*1 cup Liquid Erythritol*

*1 cup coconut oil, freshly melted and still warm*

Directions:

1. In a food processor place all nuts and chop for 1-2 minutes.

2. Add in grated coconut, almond butter, Erythritol and coconut oil. Process it for 1 minute about.

3. Cover a square bowl with parchment paper and place the mixture on top.

4. Flatten the mixture with a spatula. Place the bowl in the freezer for 4-5 hours.

5. Remove batter from the freezer, cut and serve.

*[Calories 193.62 | Total Fats 18.2g | Net Carbs: 6.64g | Protein 3.83g | Fiber 2.53g]*

# Chia Seed Cream

[Total Time: 12 HR| Serve: 4]

*Ingredients:*

*¼ cup Chia seeds*

*1 cup heavy whipping cream*

*1 cup coconut milk*

*2 Tbsp cocoa powder*

*Pure vanilla extract*

*¼ cup Erythritol sweetener*

Directions:

1. In a bowl mix the chia seeds and add the coconut milk until it combines well.

2. Add the Erythritol and whisk some more. Divide the mixture into two portions.

3. Add cocoa to one-half and mixed it nicely.

4. Pour chia seed mixture into the bowls or glasses. Keep covered in the refrigerator for 12 hours.

5. Before serving to beat the heavy whipping cream and pour over the chia seeds cream. Enjoy!

   *[Calories 341.31 | Total Fats 35.41g | Net Carbs: 7.35g | Protein 2.99g |Fiber: 1.56g]*

## Chocolate Brownies

[Total Time: 35 MIN| Serve: 10]

*Ingredients:*

*2 eggs*

*1 ½ cups almond flour*

*¼ cup coconut oil*

*½ cup cocoa powder, unsweetened*

*1 Tbsp Metamucil Fiber Powder*

*1/3 cup Natvia (or some other natural sweetener)l*

*¼ cup maple syrup*

*1 tsp baking powder*

*½ tsp salt*

Directions:

1.   Preheat oven to 350⁰F.

2.   In a bowl add in all wet ingredients and 2 Eggs. Beat the wet ingredients together using a hand mixer until a consistent mixture is formed.

3.   In a separate bowl, combine all dry ingredients. Mix the dry ingredients well. Pour the wet ingredients slowly into the dry ingredients, mixing with a hand mixer as you pour.

4.    Pour the batter into baking pan. Bake the brownies for 20 minutes.

5.    When ready, let the brownies cool. Slice brownies into slices and serve.

*[Calories 157.81 | Total Fats 13.4g | Net Carbs: 8.7g | Protein 5.4g | Fiber 2.58g]*

## Chocolate Pecan Bites

[Total Time: 3 HR| Serve: 12]

*Ingredients:*

*2 oz 100% dark chocolate*

*2.5 oz pecan halves*

*Cinnamon*

*Nutmeg*

Directions:

1.    Preheat oven to 350⁰F.

2.    Place the pecan halves on a parchment paper and bake in the oven for 6-7 minutes. When ready, let cool and set aside.

3.    Melt the dark chocolate.

4.    Dip each pecan half in the melted dark chocolate and place back on the parchment paper.

5.    Sprinkle a cinnamon and nutmeg on top of the chocolate covered pecans.

6.    Before serving place in refrigerator for 2-3 hours.

*[Calories 52.13 | Total Fats 4.96g | Net Carbs: 2.32g | Protein 0.64g |Fiber: 0.71g]*


## Hazelnuts Chocolate Cream

[Total Time: 5 MIN| Serve: 4]

*Ingredients:*

*1 cup hazelnuts halves*

*4 Tbsp unsweetened cocoa powder*

*1 tsp pure vanilla extract*

*2 Tbsp coconut oil*

*4 Tbsp granulated Stevia (or sweetener of choice)*

Directions:

1.  Place all the ingredients in your blender. Blend until smooth well.

2.  Store in the fridge for 1 hour. Serve and enjoy!

    *[Calories 302.88 | Total Fats 29.65g | Net Carbs: 9.5g | Protein 6.39g | Fiber 5.12g]*


## Instant Coffee Ice Cream

[Total Time: 20 MIN| Serve: 2]

*Ingredients:*

*1 Tbsp Instant Coffee*

*2 Tbsp Cocoa Powder*

*1 cup coconut milk*

*¼ cup heavy cream*

¼ tsp flax seeds

2 Tbsp Erythritol

15 drops liquid Nutria

Directions:

1. Add all ingredients except the flax seeds into a container of your immersion blender.

2. Blend well untiloall ingredients are incorporated well. Slowly add in flax seeds until a slightly thicker mixture is formed. Add the mass to your ice cream machine and follow manufacturer's instructions.

3. Ready! Serve!

   *[Calories 286.99 | Total Fats 29.21g | Net Carbs: 9.39g | Protein 3.18g | Fiber: 1.88 g]*

## *Jam Cookies*

[Total Time: 36 MIN| Serve: 16]

*Ingredients:*

*2 eggs*

*1 cup almond flour*

*2 Tbsp coconut flour*

*2 Tbsp sugar-free jam per taste*

*½ cup natural sweetener*

*4 tbsp coconut oil*

*½ tsp pure vanilla extract*

*½ tsp almond extract*

*1 tbsp shredded coconut*

*½ tsp baking powder*

*¼ tsp cinnamon*

*½ tsp salt*

Directions:

1.  Preheat your oven to 350⁰F. In a big bowl, combine all your dry ingredients and whisk.

2.  Add in your wet ingredients and combine well using a hand mixer or a whisk.

3.  With your hand for making the patties and place the cookies on a parchment paper-lined baking sheet. Using your finger make an indent in the middle of each cookie.

4.  Bake for about 16 minutes or until the cookies turn golden.

5.  Once ready, let the cookies cool on a wire rack and fill each indent with sugar-free jam.

6.  Before serving sprinkle some shredded coconut on top of each cookie. Enjoy!

    *[Calories 95.1 | Total Fats 8.61g | Net Carbs: 2.79g | Protein 2.71g | Fiber 1.2g]*

## Lemon Coconut Pearls

[Total Time: 15 MIN| Serve: 4]

*Ingredients:*

*3 packages of True Lemon (Crystallized Citrus for Water)*

*¼ cup shredded coconut, unsweetened*

*1 cup cream cheese*

*¼ cup granulated Stevia*

Directions:

1.  In a bowl, combine cream cheese, lemon, and Stevia. Blend well until incorporated.

2.  Once the mixture is well combined, put it back in the fridge to harden up a bit.

3.  Roll into 16 balls and dip each ball into shredded coconut. Refrigerate for several hours. Serve.

    *[Calories 216.06 | Total Fats 21.53g | Net Carbs: 3.12g | Protein 3.61g | Fiber 0.45g]*

## Lime 'n' Vanilla Cheesecake
[Total Time: 2 HR 5 MIN| Serve: 2]

*Ingredients:*

*¼ cup cream cheese, softened*

*2 Tbsp heavy cream*

*1 tsp lime juice*

*1 egg*

*1 tsp pure vanilla extract*

*2-4 Tbsp Erythritol or Stevia*

Directions:

1.  In a microwave-safe bowl combine all ingredients. Place in a microwave and cook on HIGH for 90 seconds.

2.  Every 30 seconds stir to combine the ingredients well.

3.  Transfer mixture to a bowl and refrigerate for at least 2 hours.

4.  Before serving top with whipped cream or coconut powder.

    *[Calories 140.42 | Total Fats 13.04g | Net Carbs: 1.38g | Protein 4.34g | Fiber 0.01g]*

## Chocolate Mice

[Total Time: 15 MIN| Serve: 4]

*Ingredients:*

*¼ cup of heavy cream*

*1 ¼ cup coconut cream*

*2 Tbsp of cocoa powder*

*3 Tbsp of Erythritol (or Stevia)*

*1 Tbsp pure vanilla essence*

*Shredded coconut, unsweetened*

Directions:

1.  Add coconut cream and heavy cream in the bowl and combine together using a hand mixer on low speed.

2.  Add the remaining ingredients and mix on low speed for 2-3 minutes until the mix is thick.

3.  Serve in individual ramekins sprinkled with unsweetened shredded coconut.

    *[Calories 305.19 | Total Fats 31.91g | Net Carbs: 6.97g | Protein 3.56g | Fiber 2.55g]*

## Strawberry Pudding

[Total Time: 35 MIN| Serve: 3]

*Ingredients:*

*4 egg yolks*

*2 Tbsp butter*

*¼ cup coconut flour*

*2 Tbsp heavy cream*

*¼ cup strawberries*

*¼ tsp baking powder*

*2 Tbsp coconut oil*

*2 tsp lemon juice*

*Zest 1 Lemon*

*2 Tbsp Erythritol*

*10 drops Liquid Stevia*

Directions:

1.  Preheat oven to 350⁰F.

2.  In a bowl beat the egg yolks with electric mixer until they're pale in color. Add in Erythritol and 10 drops liquid Stevia. Beat again until fully combined.

3. Add in heavy cream, lemon juice, and the zest of 1 lemon. Add the coconut and butter. Beat well until no lumps are found.

4. Sift the dry ingredients over the wet ingredients, and then mix well on a slow speed.

4. Distribute the strawberries evenly in the batter by pushing them into the top of the batter.

5. Bake for 20-25 minutes. Once finished, let cool for 5 minutes and serve.

*[Calories 258.65 | Total Fats 23.46g | Net Carbs: 9.3g | Protein 3.98g | Fiber 0.61g]*

## Kiwi Ice Cream

[Total Time: 8 HR 15 MIN| Serve: 6]

*Ingredients:*

*3 egg yolks*

*1 ½ cup Kiwi, pureed*

*1 cup heavy cream*

*1/3 cup Erythritol*

*½ tsp pure vanilla extract*

*1/8 tsp chia seeds*

Directions:

1. In a saucepan heat up the heavy cream. Add erythritol and simmer until the erythritol has dissolved.

2.  Beat 3 egg yolks in a medium sized mixing bowl with an electric mixer. Add in hot cream mixture, 1 tsp at a time to the eggs while beating. Add in some pure vanilla extract and mix. Add in 1/8 tsp. of chia seeds.

3.  Once the ingredients are combined, put your bowl into the freezer and let it chill for 1-2 hours, stirring twice.

4.  In a meanwhile puree the kiwi no more than 1-2 seconds. When the ice cream is getting a thicker, about 1 hour in add the kiwi mixture to the cream and mix well.

5.  Let the kiwi ice cream to chill at least 6-8 hours. Serve in chilled glasses.

    *[Calories 192.47 | Total Fats 17.2g | Net Carbs: 8.13g | Protein 2.69g | Fiber 1.46g]*

## Avocado Lime Sorbet
[Total Time: 3 HR 15 MIN| Serve: 6]

*Ingredients:*

*1 cup coconut milk*

*2 avocados, sliced vertically into 5 pieces*

*¼ mint leaves, chopped*

*¼ cup powdered Erythritol*

*2 limes, juiced*

*¼ tsp liquid Stevia*

Directions:

1. Place avocado pieces on foil and squeeze the ½ lime juice over the tops.

2. Place avocado in the freezer for at least 3 hours.

3. Using a spice grinder, powder Erythritol.

4. In a pan, bring coconut milk to a boil.

5. Zest the 2 limes you have while coconut milk is heating up. Add lime zest and continue to let the milk reduce in volume.

6. Remove and place the coconut milk into a container and store in the freezer.

7. Chop mint leaves. Remove avocados from the freezer.

8. Add avocado, mint leaves, and juice from lime into the food processor. Pulse until a chunky consistency is achieved.

9. Pour coconut milk mixture over the avocados in the food processor. Add Liquid Stevia to this.

10. Pulse mixture together about 2-3 minutes.

11. Return to freezer to freeze, or serve immediately!

    *[Calories 184.18 | Total Fats 17.26g | Net Carbs: 9.65g | Protein 1.95g | Fiber 4.59g]*

## *Morning Zephyr Cake*

[Total Time: 40 MIN| Serve: 8]

*Ingredients:*

*3 Tbsp coconut oil*

*2 Tbsp grounded flax seeds*

*8 Tbsp almonds, grounded*

*1 cup Greek Yogurt*

*1 Tbsp cocoa powder for dusting*

*1 cup heavy whipping cream*

*1 tsp Baking Powder*

*1 tsp Baking Soda*

*1 tsp pure vanilla essence*

*1 pinch pink salt*

*1 cup Stevia or Erythritol sweetener*

Directions:

1. Pre-heat the oven to 350$^0$F degrees.

2. In the blender first add the grounded almonds, grounded flax seeds, and the baking powder and soda. Blend for a minute.

3. Add the salt, coconut oil and blend some more. Add the sweetener and blend for 2-3 minutes.

4. Add the Greek yogurt and blend for a minute or so, until a fine consistency is reached.

5. Take out the batter in a bowl and add the vanilla essence, and mix with a light hand.

6. Grease the baking dish and drop the batter in it.

7. Bake for 30 minutes. Let cool on a wire rack. Serve.

*[Calories 199.84 | Total Fats 20.69g | Net Carbs: 3.22g | Protein 2.56g | Fiber 1.17g]*

## *Peanut Butter Balls*

[Total Time: 22 MIN| Serve: 16]

*Ingredients:*

*2 eggs*

*2 ½ cup of peanut butter*

*½ cup shredded coconut (unsweetened)*

*½ cup of Xylitol*

*1 Tbsp of pure vanilla extract*

Directions:

1. Preheat oven to 320⁰F.

2. Mix all ingredients together by your hands.

3. After the ingredients are thoroughly mixed, roll into heaped tbsp sized balls and press into a baking tray lined with baking paper.

4. Bake in preheated oven for 12 minutes.

5. When ready, let cool on a wire rack.

6. Serve and enjoy.

*[Calories 254.83 | Total Fats 21.75g | Net Carbs: 8.31g | Protein 10.98g | Fiber 2.64g]*

## Pecan Flax Seed Blondies
[Total Time: 40 MIN| Serve: 16]

*Ingredients:*

*3 eggs*

*2 ¼ cups pecans, roasted*

*3 Tbsp heavy cream*

*1 Tbsp salted caramel syrup*

*½ cup flax seeds, ground*

*¼ cup butter, melted*

*¼ cup erythritol, powdered*

*10 drops Liquid Stevia*

*1 tsp baking powder*

*1 pinch salt*

Directions:

1. Preheat oven to 350°F.
2. In a baking pan roast pecan for 10 minutes.
3. Grind ½ cup flax seeds in a spice grinder. Place flax seed powder in a bowl. Grind Erythritol in a spice grinder until powdered. Set in the same bowl as the flax seed meal.

4.  Place 2/3 of roasted pecans in food processor and process until a smooth nut butter is formed.

5.  Add eggs, liquid Stevia, salted caramel syrup, and a pinch of salt to the flax seed mixture. Mix well. Add pecan butter to the batter and mix again.

6.  Crush the remaining roasted pecans into chunks.

7.  Add crushed pecans and 1/4 cup melted butter into the batter.

8.  Mix batter well and then add heavy cream and baking powder. Mix everything together well.

9.  Place the batter into baking tray and bake for 20 minutes.

10. Let cool for about 10 minutes.

11. Cut into square and serve.

    *[Calories 180.45 | Total Fats 18.23g | Net Carbs: 3.54g | Protein 3.07g | Fiber 1.78g]*

## Chocolate Chip Ice Cream

[Total Time: 35 MIN| Serve: 3]

*Ingredients:*

*½ tsp Peppermint extract*

*1 cup heavy cream*

*1 cup cheese cream*

*1 tsp pure vanilla extract*

*1 tsp Liquid Stevia extract*

*100% Dark Chocolate for topping*

Directions:

1. Place ice cream bowl in the freezer.
2. In a metal bowl, add all ingredients except chocolate and whisk well.
3. Put back in the freezer for 5 minutes.
6. Set up ice cream maker and add liquid.
7. Before serving, top the ice cream with chocolate shavings. Serve.

   *[Calories 286.66 | Total Fats 29.96g | Net Carbs: 2.7g | Protein 2.6g]*

## *Low Carb Coconut Waffles*
[Total Time: 20 MIN| Serve: 8]

*Ingredients:*

*1 cup coconut flour*

*½ cup heavy (whipping) cream*

*5 eggs*

*¼ tsp pink salt*

*¼ tsp baking soda*

*¼ cup coconut milk*

*2 tsp Yacon Syrup*

*2 Tbsp coconut oil (melted)*

Directions:

1.  In a large bowl add the eggs and beat with an electric hand mixer for 30 seconds.

2.  Add the heavy (whipping) cream and coconut oil into the eggs while you are still mixing. Add the coconut milk, coconut flour, pink salt and baking soda. Mix with the hand mixer for 45 seconds on low speed. Set aside.

3.  Heat up your waffle maker well and make the waffles according to your manufactures specifications.

4.  Serve hot.

    *[Calories 169.21 | Total Fats 12.6g | Net Carbs: 9.97g | Protein 4.39g | Fiber 0.45g]*

## *Raspberry Chocolate Ice Cream*

[Total Time: 15 MIN| Serve: 4]

*Ingredients:*

*½ cup 100% dark chocolate, chopped*

*¼ cup of heavy cream*

*½ cup cream cheese, softened*

*2 Tbsp sugar-free Raspberry Syrup*

*¼ up Erythritol*

Directions:

1.  In a double boiler melt chopped chocolate and the cream cheese. Add the Erythritol sweetener and continue to stir. Remove from heat, let cool and set aside.

2.  When the cream has cooled add in heavy cream and Raspberry syrup and stir well.

3.  Pour cream in a bowls or glasses and serve. Keep refrigerated.

    *[Calories 157.67 | Total Fats 13.51g | Net Carbs: 7.47g | Protein 1.95g | Fiber 1g]*

## Raw Cacao Hazelnut Cookies
[Total Time: 6 HR| Serve: 24]

*Ingredients:*

*2 cups almond flour*

*1 cup chopped hazelnuts*

*½ cup cacao powder*

*½ cup ground flax*

*3 Tbsp coconut oil (melted)*

*1/3 cup water*

*1/3 cup Erythritol*

*¼ tsp liquid Stevia*

Directions:

1.  In a bowl, mix flax and almond flour, cacao powder.

2.  Stir in oil, water, agave, and vanilla. When it is well combined, stir in chopped hazelnuts.

3.  Form into balls, press flat with palms and place on dehydrator screens.

4.  Dehydrate one hour at 145, then reduce to 116 and dehydrate for at least five hours.

5.  Serve and enjoy.

    *[Calories 181.12 | Total Fats 15.69g | Net Carbs: 8.75g | Protein 4.46g | Fiber: 3.45 g]*


## *Sinless Pumpkin Cheesecake Muffins*
[Total Time: 15 MIN| Serve: 6]

*Ingredients:*

*½ cup pureed pumpkin*

*1 tsp pumpkin pie spice*

*½ up pecans, finely ground*

*½ cup cream cheese*

*1 Tbsp coconut oil*

*½ tsp pure vanilla extract*

*¼ tsp pure Yacon Syrup or Erythritol*


Directions:

1. Prepare a muffin tin with liners.

2. Place a few ground pecans into every muffin tin and make a thin crust.

3. In a bowl, blend sweetener, spices, vanilla, coconut and the pumpkin puree. Add in the cream cheese and beat until the mixture is well combined.

4. Scoop about two tbsp of filling mixture on top of each crust, and smooth the edges.

5. Pop in the freezer for about 45 minutes.

6. Remove from the muffin tin and let sit for 10 minutes. Serve.

   *[Calories 157.34 | Total Fats 15.52g | Net Carbs: 3.94g | Protein 2.22g | Fiber: 1.51g]*

## *Sour Hazelnuts Biscuits with Arrowroot Tea*
[Total Time: 50 MIN| Serve: 12]

*Ingredients:*

*1 egg*

*½ cup hazelnuts*

*3 Tbsp of coconut oil*

*2 cups almond flour*

*2 Tbsp of arrowroot tea*

*2 tsp ginger*

*1 Tbsp cocoa powder*

*½ cup grapefruit juice*

1 orange peel from a half orange

½ tsp baking soda

1 pinch of salt

Directions:

1. Preheat oven to 360°F.

2. Make arrowroot tea and let it cool.

3. In a food processor blend the hazelnuts. Add the remaining ingredients and continue blending until mixed well. With your hands form cookies with the batter.

4. Put the cookies on baking parchment paper, and bake for 30-35 minutes. When ready, remove the tray from the oven and let cool.

5. Serve warm or cold.

[Calories 224.08 | Total Fats 20.17g | Net Carbs: 8.06g | Protein 6.36g | Fiber 3.25 g]

## Tartar Keto Cookies
[Total Time: 35 MIN| Serve: 8]

Ingredients:

3 eggs

1/8 tsp cream of tartar

1/3 cup cream cheese

1/8 tsp salt

Some oil for greasing

Directions:

1. Preheat oven to 300⁰F.

2. Line the cookie sheet with parchment paper and grease with some oil.

3. Separate eggs from the egg yolks. Set both in different mixing bowls.

4. With an electric hand mixer, start beating the egg whites until super bubbly. Add in cream of tartar and beat until stiff peaks form.

5. In the egg yolk bowl, add in cream cheese and some salt. Beat until the egg yolks are pale yellow.

6. Merge the egg whites into the cream cheese mixture.

7. Stir well.

8. Make cookies and place on the cookie sheet.

9. Bake for about 30-40 minutes. When ready, let them cool on a wire rack and serve.

*[Calories 59.99 | Total Fats 5.09g | Net Carbs: 0.56g | Protein 2.93g]*

## *Wild Strawberries Ice Cream*
[Total Time: 5 MIN| Serve: 4]

*Ingredients:*

*½ cup wild strawberries*

*1/3 cup cream cheese*

*1 cup heavy cream*

*1 Tbsp lemon juice*

*1 tsp pure vanilla extract*

*1/3 cup of your favorite sweetener*

*Ice cubes*

Directions:

1.  Place all ingredients in a blender. Blend until all incorporate well.

2.  Refrigerate for 2-3 hour before serving.

    *[Calories 176.43 | Total Fats 17.69g | Net Carbs: 3.37g | Protein 1.9g | Fiber 0.39g]*

## *Mini Lemon Cheesecakes*
[Total Time: 5 MIN| Serve: 6]

*Ingredients:*

*1 tbsp lemon zest, grated*

*1 tsp lemon juice*

*½ tsp stevia powder or (Truvia)*

*1/4 cup coconut oil, softened*

*4 tbsp unsalted butter, softened*

*4 ounces cream cheese (heavy cream)*

Directions:

1.  Blend all ingredients together with a hand mixer or blender until smooth and creamy.
2.  Prepare a cupcake or muffin tin with 6 paper liners.
3.  Pour mixture into prepared tin and place in freezer for 2-3 hours or until firm.
4.  Sprinkle cups with additional lemon zest. Or try using chopped nuts or shredded, unsweetened coconut.

    *[Calories 213 | Total Fats 23g | Net Carbs: 0.7g | Protein 1.5g | Fiber: 0.1 g]*

## Chocolate Layered Coconut Cups
[Total Time: 55 MIN| Serve: 10]

*Ingredients:*

*Bottom Layer:*

*½ cup unsweetened, shredded coconut*

*3 tbsp powdered sweeteners such as Splenda or Truvia*

*½ cup coconut butter*

*½ cup coconut oil*

*Top Layer:*

*1 ½ ounces cocoa butter*

*1-ounce unsweetened chocolate*

¼ *cup cocoa powder*

½ *tsp vanilla extract*

¼ *cup powdered sweetener such as Splenda or Truvia*

Directions:

1. Prepare a mini-muffin pan with 20 mini paper liners.
   For the bottom layer:

2. Combine coconut oil and coconut butter in a small saucepan over low heat.

3. Stir until smooth and melted then add the shredded coconut and powdered sweetener until well combined.

4. Divide the mixture among prepared mini muffin cups and place in the refrigerator for 30 minutes.

5. For the top layer:
   Combine cocoa butter and unsweetened chocolate together in double boiler or a bowl set over a pan of simmering water. Stir until melted.

6. Stir in the powdered sweetener, then the cocoa powder and mix until smooth.

7. Remove from heat and stir in the vanilla extract.

8. Spoon chocolate mixture over coconut candies and let them set for 15 minutes.

9. Serve and enjoy.

[Calories 300| Total Fats 27g | Net Carbs: 14.5g | Protein 2g | Fiber: 3.9g]

## Pumpkin Pie Chocolate Cups

*[Total Time: 45 MIN | Serve: 18]*

*Ingredients:*

*For the crust:*

*3.5 ounces extra dark chocolate - 85% cocoa solids or more*

*2 tbsp coconut oil*

*For the pie:*

*½ cup coconut butter*

*¼ cup coconut oil*

*2 tsp pumpkin pie spice mix*

*½ cup unsweetened pumpkin puree*

*2 tbsp healthy low-carb sweetener*

*Optional: 15-20 drops liquid stevia for added sweetness*

Directions:

1. Place the chocolate and coconut oil in a double boiler or a glass bowl on top of a small saucepan filled with simmering water. Once completely melted, remove from the heat and set aside.

2. Prepare a mini muffin tin with 18 paper liners.

3. Fill each of the 18 mini muffin cups with 2 tsp of the chocolate mixture.

4. Place the chocolate in the refrigerator for 10 minutes.

5. Place the coconut butter, coconut oil, sweetener and pumpkin spice mix into a bowl and melt just like you did the chocolate.

6. Add the pumpkin puree and mix until smooth and well combined.

7. Remove the muffin cups from the fridge and add a heaping tsp of the pumpkin & coconut mixture into every cup.

8. Place back in the refrigerator and let it sit for 30 minutes.

9. When done, keep refrigerated. Coconut oil and butter get very soft at room temperature.

10. Store in the refrigerator.

11. Serve and enjoy.

    *[Calories 92| Total Fats 9.1g | Net Carbs: 3.4g | Protein 0.7g | Fiber: 1.6g]*


## *Fudgy Cake*

[Total Time: 3 HR 20 MIN| Serve: 10]

*Ingredients:*

*1 ½ cups almond flour*

*¼ cup whey protein powder (chocolate, vanilla, and unflavored all work fine)*

*3/4  cup sugar substitute  such as Swerve or Truvia*

*2/3 cup cocoa powder*

*2 tsp baking powder*

*¼  tsp sea salt*

*½ cup butter, melted*

*4 large eggs*

*3/4 cup almond or coconut milk,  unsweetened*

*1 tsp vanilla extract*

*½ cup chopped dark chocolate, 85% cocoa or higher*

*Whipped cream topping  (optional):*

*½ cup heavy whipping cream*

*2 tbsp sugar substitute*

Directions:

1.  Grease the insert of a 6-quart slow cooker well with butter or coconut oil.

2.  In a medium bowl, whisk together almond flour, sugar substitute, cocoa powder, whey protein powder, baking powder, and salt.

3.  Stir in butter, eggs, almond milk and vanilla extract until well combined, then fold in the chopped dark chocolate.

4.  Pour into the greased slow cooker and cook on low for 2.5 to 3 hours. It will be gooey and like a pudding cake at 2.5 hours and little more cake-like at 3 hours.

5.  Turn slow cooker off and let cool for 20 to 30 minutes. Cut into pieces and serve warm.

6.  Best when served with freshly whipped cream. To make this, mix the whipping cream and sugar substitute together with your stand mixer, or a hand mixer. Continue mixing until soft peaks form.

    *[Calories 313 | Total Fats 26g | Net Carbs: 14g | Protein 10g | Fiber: 4.7g]*


## Easy Sticky Chocolate Fudge
[Total Time: 25 MIN| Serve: 12]

*Ingredients:*

*1 cup coconut oil, softened*

*¼ cup coconut milk (full fat, from a can)*

*¼ cup cocoa powder*

*1 tsp vanilla extract*

*½ tsp sea salt*

*1-3 drops liquid stevia*


Directions:

1.  With a hand mixer or stand mixer, whip the softened coconut oil and coconut milk together until smooth and glossy. About 6 minutes on high.

2.  Add the cocoa powder, vanilla extract, sea salt, and one drop of liquid stevia to the bowl and mix on low

until combined. Increase speed once everything is combined and mix for one minute. Taste fudge and adjust sweetness by adding additional liquid stevia, if desired.

3. Prepare a 9"x4" loaf pan by lining it with parchment paper.
4. Pour fudge into loaf pan and place in freezer for about 15, until just set.
5. Remove fudge and cut into 1" x 1" pieces.
6. Store in an airtight container in the refrigerator.

*[Calories 173 | Total Fats 19g | Net Carbs: 1.3g | Protein 0.4g | Fiber: 0.6g]*

## *Raspberry 'n' Coconut Fat Bombs*
[Total Time: 15 MIN| Serve: 12]

*Ingredients:*

*½ cup coconut butter*

*½ cup coconut oil*

*½ cup freeze dried raspberries*

*½ cup unsweetened shredded coconut*

*¼ powdered sugar substitute such as Swerve or Truvia*

Directions:

1. Line an 8"x8" pan with parchment paper.

2. In a food processor, coffee grinder, or blender, pulse the dried raspberries into a fine powder.

3. In a saucepan over medium heat, combine the coconut butter, coconut oil, coconut, and sweetener. Stir until melted and well combined.

4. Remove pan from heat and stir in raspberry powder.

5. Pour mixture into the pan and refrigerate or freeze for several hours, or overnight.

6. Cut into 12 pieces and serve.

*[Calories 189 | Total Fats 17.8g | Net Carbs: 7.9g | Protein 1.1g | Fiber: 3.1g]*

## Strawberry Cheesecake Ice Cream Cups
[Total Time: 10 MIN| Serve: 12]

*Ingredients:*

*½ strawberries, fresh or frozen, mashed well*

*¾ cup cream cheese, softened*

*¼ cup coconut oil, softened*

*10-15 drops liquid stevia*

*1 tsp vanilla extract*

Directions:

1. Combine all ingredients in a medium-sized bowl and mix with a hand mixer until smooth and creamy.

Can also be done in a food processor or high-speed blender.)

2. Spoon the mixture into mini muffin silicon molds or small candy molds. Place in the freezer for about 2 hours or until set.

3. When done, unmold the fat bombs and place into a container. Keep in the freezer and enjoy anytime!

*[Calories 91 | Total Fats 9.6g | Net Carbs: 0.5g | Protein 1.1g]*

# Peppermint Patties

[Total Time: 10 MIN| Serve: 12]

*Ingredients:*

*¾ cup melted coconut butter*

*¼ cup finely shredded, unsweetened coconut*

*2 tbsp cacao powder*

*3 tbsp coconut oil, melted*

*½ tsp pure peppermint extract*

Directions:

1. Mix together melted coconut butter, shredded coconut, 1 tbsp of coconut oil and peppermint extract

2. Pour coconut butter mixture into mini muffin tins that have been lined with paper liners. Fill halfway.

3. Place in refrigerator and allow to harden for about 15 minutes.

4. Mix together 2 tbsp coconut oil and cacao powder.

5. Remove muffin tin from the refrigerator and top each one with chocolate mixture.

6. Return to refrigerator until the chocolate has set.

7. When ready to eat, simply set the peppermint patty cups on the counter for about 5 minutes and unmold from muffin tin.

*[Calories 137 | Total Fats 22.6g | Net Carbs: 4.4g | Protein 1.3g | Fiber: 3g]*


## Buttery Pecan Delights
[Total Time: 15 MIN| Serve: 2]

*Ingredients:*

*8 pecan halves*

*1 tbsp unsalted butter, softened*

*2 ounces neufchâtel cheese*

*1 tsp orange zest, finely grated*

*Pinch of sea salt*

Directions:

1. Toast the pecans at 350 degrees F for 5-10 minutes, check often to prevent burning.

2. Mix the butter, neufchâtel cheese, and orange zest until smooth and creamy.

3. Spread the butter mixture between the cooled pecan halves and sandwich together.

4. Sprinkle with sea salt and enjoy.

   *[Calories 129 | Total Fats 12.8g | Net Carbs: 1.2g | Protein 3g | Fiber: 02g]*


## Fudge Oh So Chocolate
[Total Time: 20 MIN| Serve: 12]

*Ingredients:*

*1 cup coconut oil, softened*

*¼ cup coconut milk (full fat, from a can)*

*½ tsp sea salt*

*1-3 drops liquid stevia*

*¼ cup cocoa powder*

*1 tsp vanilla extract*


Directions:

1. With a hand mixer or stand mixer, whip the softened coconut oil and coconut milk together until smooth and glossy. About 6 minutes on high.

2. Add the cocoa powder, vanilla extract, sea salt, and one drop of liquid stevia to the bowl and mix on low until combined. Increase speed once everything is combined and mix for one minute. Taste fudge and adjust sweetness by adding additional liquid stevia, if desired.

3. Prepare a 9"x4" loaf pan by lining it with parchment paper.

4. Pour fudge into loaf pan and place in freezer for about 15, ountil just set.

5. Remove fudge and cut into 1" x 1" pieces.

6. Store in an airtight container in the refrigerator.

   *[Calories 173 | Total Fats 19.6g | Net Carbs: 1.3g | Protein 0.4g | Fiber: 0.6g]*

## Cinna-Bun Balls

[Total Time: 15 MIN| Serve: 10]

*Ingredients:*

*1 cup coconut butter*

*1 tsp vanilla extract*

*1 cup full-fat coconut milk (from a can)*

*1 cup unsweetened coconut shreds*

*½ tsp cinnamon*

*½ tsp nutmeg*

*1 tsp sugar substitute such as Splenda*

Directions:

1. Combine all ingredients except the shredded coconut together in double boiler or a bowl set over a pan of simmering water. Stir until everything is melted and combined.

2. Remove bowl from heat and place in the fridge until the mixture has firmed up and can be rolled into balls.

3. Form the mixture into 1" balls, a small cookie scoop is helpful for doing this.

4. Roll each ball in the shredded coconut until well coated.

5. Serve and enjoy! Store in the fridge.

*[Calories 280 | Total Fats 26.6g | Net Carbs: 9.9g | Protein 3g | Fiber: 6.2g]*

## *Vanilla Mousse Cups*

[Total Time: 15 MIN| Serve: 6]

*Ingredients:*

*8 ounces (1 block) cream cheese, softened*

*½ cup sugar substitute such as Swerve or Truvia (Stevia)*

*1 ½ tsp vanilla extract*

*Dash of sea salt*

*½ cup heavy whipping cream*

Directions:

1.   Add the first four ingredients to a food processor or blender.

2.   Blend until combined.

3.   With blender running, slowly add the heavy cream.

4.   Continue to blend until thickened, about 1-2 minutes. Consistency should be mousse-like.

5.   Prepare a cupcake or muffin tin with 6 paper liners and portion the mixture into the cups.

6.   Chill in the fridge until set and enjoy!

*[Calories 170 | Total Fats 16.9g | Net Carbs: 1.6g | Protein 3.1g]*


## Rich 'n' Creamy Fat Bomb Ice Cream
[Total Time: 20 MIN| Serve: 5]

Ingredients:

*4 whole pastured eggs*

*4 yolks from pastured eggs*

*⅓ Cup melted cocoa butter*

*⅓ Cup melted coconut oil*

*15-20 drops liquid stevia*

*⅓ Cup cocoa powder*

*¼ cup MCT oil*

*2 tsp pure vanilla extract*

*8-10 ice cubes*

Directions:

1. Add all ingredients but the ice cubes into the jug of your high-speed blender. Blend on high for 2 minutes, until creamy.

2. While the blender is running, remove the top portion of the lid and drop in 1 ice cube at a time, allowing the blender to run about 10 seconds between each ice cube.

3. Once all of the ice has been added, pour the cold mixture into a 9×5" loaf pan and place in the freezer. Set the timer for 30 minutes before taking out to stir. Repeat this process for 2-3 hours, until desired consistency is met.

4. Serve immediately. Top with chopped nuts or shaved dark chocolate, if desired.

5. Store covered in the freezer for up to a week.

   *[Calories 448 | Total Fats 48.1g | Net Carbs: 4.1g | Protein 7.6g | Fiber 1.7g]*

## English Toffee Treats

[Total Time: 10 MIN| Serve: 24]

*Ingredients:*

*1 cup coconut oil*

2 tbsp butter

½ block cream cheese, softened

3/4 tbsp cocoa powder

½ cup creamy, natural peanut butter

3 tbsp Davinci Gourmet Sugar-Free English Toffee Syrup

Directions:

1. Combine all ingredients in a saucepan over medium heat.

2. Stir until everything is smooth, melted, and combined.

3. Pour mixture into small candy molds or mini muffin tins lined with paper liners.

4. Freeze or refrigerate until set and enjoy!

5. Store in an airtight container in the fridge.

   *[Calories 125 | Total Fats 13.4g | Net Carbs: 1.1g | Protein 1.3g]*

## Fudgy Peanut Butter Squares

[Total Time: 10 MIN| Serve: 12]

Ingredients:

1 cup all natural creamy peanut butter

1 cup coconut oil

¼ cup unsweetened vanilla almond milk

a pinch of coarse sea salt

1 tsp vanilla extract

*2 tsp liquid stevia (optional)*

Directions:

1. In a microwave-safe bowl, soften the peanut butter and coconut oil together. (About 1 minute on med-low heat.)
2. Combine the softened peanut butter and coconut oil with the remaining ingredients into a blender or food processor.
3. Blend until thoroughly combined.
4. Pour into a 9X4" loaf pan that has been lined with parchment paper.
5. Refrigerate until set. About 2 hours.
6. Enjoy.

*[Calories 292 | Total Fats 28.9g | Net Carbs: 4.1g | Protein 6g | Fiber 1.4g]*

## Lemon Squares 'n' Coconut Cream
[Total Time: 1 HR 5 MIN| Serve: 8]

*Ingredients:*

*Base:*

*3/4 cup coconut flakes*

*2 Tbsp coconut oil*

*1 Tbsp ground almonds*

*Cream:*

5 eggs

½ lemon juice

1 Tbsp coconut flour

½ cup Stevia sweetener

Directions:

1.  For the base
2.  Preheat oven to 360⁰F.
3.  In a bowl put all base ingredients and with clean hands mix everything well until soft.
4.  With coconut oil grease a rectangle oven dish. Pour dough into a baking pan. Bake for 15 minutes until golden brown. Set aside to cool.
5.  For the cream
6.  In a bowl or blender, whisk together: eggs, lemon juice, coconut flour, and sweetener. Pour over the baked caked evenly.
7.  Put the pan in the oven and bake 20 minutes more.
8.  When ready refrigerate for at least 6 hours. Cut into cubes and serve.

    *[Calories 129 | Total Fats 15g | Net Carbs: 1.4g | Protein 5g | Fiber 2.25g]*

## *Rich Almond Butter Cake 'n' Chocolate Sauce*

[Total Time: 10 MIN| Serve: 12]

## Ingredients:

*1 cup almond butter or soaked almonds*

*¼ cup almond milk, unsweetened*

*1 cup coconut oil*

*2 tsp liquid Stevia sweetener to taste*

*Topping: Chocolate Sauce*

*4 Tbsp cocoa powder, unsweetened*

*2 Tbsp almond butter*

*2 Tbsp Stevia sweetener*

## Directions:

1.  Melt the coconut oil in room temperature.
2.  Add all ingredients in a bowl and blend well until combined.
3.  Pour the almond butter mixture into a parchment lined platter.
4.  Place in refrigerator for 3 hours.
5.  In a bowl, whisk all topping ingredients together. Pour over the almond cake after it's been set. Cut into cubes and serve.

    *[Calories 273 | Total Fats 23.3g | Net Carbs: 2.4g | Protein 5.8g | Fiber 2g]*

## *Peanut Butter Cake Covered in Chocolate Sauce*
[Total Time: 10 MIN| Serve: 12]

*Ingredients:*

*1 cup peanut butter*

*¼ cup almond milk, unsweetened*

*1 cup coconut oil*

*2 tsp liquid Stevia sweetener to taste*

*Topping: Chocolate Sauce*

*2 Tbsp coconut oil, melted*

*4 Tbsp cocoa powder, unsweetened*

*2 Tbsp Stevia sweetener*

Directions:

1. In a microwave bowl mix coconut oil and peanut butter; melt in a microwave for 1-2 minutes.
2. Add this mixture to your blender; add in the rest of the ingredients and blend well until combined.
3. Pour the peanut mixture into a parchment lined loaf pan or platter.
4. Refrigerate for about 3 hours; the longer, the better.
5. In a bowl, whisk all topping ingredients together. Pour over the peanut candy after it's been set. Cut into cubes and serve.

[Calories 273 | Total Fats 27g | Net Carbs: 2.4g | Protein 6g | Fiber 2g]

# Snacks

## Greek-Style Fat Bomb Balls

[Total Time: 15 MIN| Serve: 5]

Ingredients:

½ cup Cream cheese softened

¼ cup Butter softened

3 tsp freshly chopped or dry herbs (any combination of basil, thyme, oregano and/or parsley works great)

4 pieces sun-dried tomatoes, drained

4 Kalamata olives, pitted and chopped

2 cloves garlic, crushed

Freshly ground black pepper

¼ tsp Sea salt

5 tbsp Parmesan cheese, finely grated

Directions:

1. Mash the butter and cream cheese together with a fork and mix until well combined. Mix in the chopped sun-dried tomatoes and chopped Kalamata olives.

2. Add the freshly chopped herbs (or dried), crushed garlic and season with pepper and salt.

3.  Mix well and place in refrigerator for 20-30 minutes.

4.  Remove the cheese mixture from refrigerator and make 5 balls.

5.  Place the grated parmesan cheese in a dish.

6.  Coat each ball in the grated parmesan cheese and place on a plate.

7.  Serve immediately or store in refrigerator in an airtight container.

    *[Calories 195 | Total Fats 19.1g | Net Carbs: 2.7g | Protein 4.1g | Fiber 0.6g]*

## Bacon 'n' Onion Cookie Bites

[Total Time: 25 MIN| Serve: 12]

*Ingredients:*

*1 ½ cups Almond Flour*

*1/3 cup Flax meal*

*1 tbsp Psyllium husk powder*

*1 tbsp Onion powder*

*1 large egg*

*4 slices bacon, cooked until crispy and crumbled*

*½ tsp Sea salt*

*Freshly ground pepper*

Directions:

1. Place all of the dry ingredients into a bowl and mix until well combined.

2. Add the egg and mix well using your hands.

3. Add the crumbled bacon to the dough. Process well using your hands.

4. Using your hand, make 12 equal balls and place them on a baking sheet lined with parchment paper.

5. Use a fork to press and flatten the dough.

6. Place in the oven and bake for 10-12 minutes.

7. When done, the cookies should be golden brown. Remove from oven and cool on a wire rack.

8. Store in a container.

9. Serve and enjoy.

   *[Calories 151 | Total Fats 12.3g | Net Carbs: 6.1g | Protein 7.3g | Fiber: 3.9g]*

## Guacamole 'n' Bacon Fat Bombs

[Total Time: 30 MIN| Serve: 6]

*Ingredients:*

*1 large avocado, halved and peeled*

*¼ cup Butter softened*

*2 cloves garlic, crushed*

*1 tsp Crushed red pepper*

*½ small white onion, diced*

1 tbsp Fresh lime juice

Freshly ground black pepper

¼ tsp Sea salt

4 large slices bacon

2 tbsp Bacon grease, reserved from cooking


Directions:
1. Preheat the oven to 375⁰F.
2. Line a baking tray with parchment paper. Lay the bacon strips out flat on the parchment paper, leaving space so they don't overlap.
3. Place the tray in the oven and cook for about 10-15 minutes until golden brown and crisp.
4. When done, remove from the oven and set aside to cool down.
5. Place the avocado, butter, crushed red pepper, garlic and lime juice into a bowl and season with pepper and salt.
6. Mash using masher until well combined.
7. Add the diced onion and mix well.
8. Pour in the 2 tbsp of reserved bacon grease and mix well.
9. Cover with foil and place in the refrigerator for 20-30 minutes.

10. Chop the bacon into pieces and place in a dish.

11. Remove the guacamole mixture from refrigerator and make 6 balls.

12. Coat each ball in the bacon crumbles and place on a tray.

13. Serve immediately or store in the refrigerator in an airtight container for up to 5 days.

*[Calories 210 | Total Fats 19.6g | Net Carbs: 4.2g | Protein 5.6g | Fiber: 2.5g]*

## *Bacon and Egg Fat Bombs*

[Total Time: 30 MIN| Serve: 6]

*Ingredients:*

*2 large eggs, hard-boiled, peel and quarter*

*¼ cup Butter softened*

*2 tbsp Mayonnaise*

*Freshly ground black pepper*

*½ tsp Sea salt*

*4 large slices bacon*

*2 tbsp Bacon grease, reserved from cooking*

Directions:

1. Preheat the oven to 375⁰F.

2. Line a baking tray with parchment paper.

3.  Lay the bacon strips out flat on the baking paper, leaving space so they don't overlap.
4.  Place the tray in the oven and cook for about 10-15 minutes until golden brown.
5.  When done, remove from the oven and set aside to cool down.
6.  Cut butter into pieces and add the quartered eggs. Mash with a fork.
7.  Add the mayonnaise, season with pepper and salt and mix well.
8.  Pour in the bacon grease and mix well.
9.  Place in the refrigerator for 20-30 minutes.
10. Chop the bacon into pieces and place in a dish.
11. Remove the egg mixture from refrigerator and make 6 balls.
12. Serve immediately or store in refrigerator in an airtight container for up to 5 days.

*[Calories 179 | Total Fats 16.3g | Net Carbs: 1.5g | Protein 6.9g]*

## *Simple Parmesan Crisps*

[Total Time: 25 MIN| Serve: 4]

*Ingredients:*

*1 cup Parmesan cheese*

*4 tbsp Coconut Flour*

*2 tsp Rosemary, oregano or any herbs of choice, dried or fresh*

Directions:

1. Preheat the oven to 3500F.
2. In a small bowl, mix the coconut flour and grated parmesan cheese.
3. Scoop a tsp of the cheese mixture onto a baking tray lined with parchment paper leaving a small gap between each.
4. Place in preheated oven and cook for 10-15 minutes or until golden brown.
5. Remove from the oven and let the crisps cool down before you remove them from the baking tray.
6. Serve and enjoy.

   *[Calories 144 | Total Fats 7.5g | Net Carbs: 8.9g | Protein 9.6g |Fiber: 5.1g]*

## Mini Pizza Bombs

[Total Time: 10 MIN| Serve: 6]

*Ingredients:*

*14 slices Italian sausages*

*8 pitted black olives*

*¾ cup Cream cheese*

*2 Tbsp fresh basil, chopped*

2 Tbsp pesto

Salt and pepper to taste

Directions:

1. Dice pitted Kalamata olives and pepperoni into small pieces.

2. Mix together cream cheese, basil, and pesto.

3. Add the olives and sausage slices into the cream cheese and mix again.

4. Form into balls and garnish with pepperoni, basil, and olive. Ready!!

   [Calories 261 | Total Fats 23.43g | Net Carbs: 1g | Protein 10.4g |Fiber: 0.7g]

## Cheesy Bacon Fat Bombs
[Total Time: 15 MIN| Serve: 24]

Ingredients:

8 strips cooked crispy bacon, crumbled

1 cup cream cheese, softened

½ cup butter

4 tsp bacon fat

4 Tbsp coconut oil

¼ cup Splenda to taste

Directions:

1. In a microwave dish, combine all ingredients and melt slowly in the microwave until smooth. Set aside some crumbled bacon,

2. Pour into a dish or pan and place in the freezer until firm, about 30 minutes.

3. Before serving, remove from freezer, sprinkle with more crumbled bacon, slice and serve.

   *[Calories 151 | Total Fats 15.9g | Net Carbs: 0.3g | Protein 0g]*


## Smoked Turkey, Blue Cheese Eggs

[Total Time: 20 MIN| Serve: 6]

*Ingredients:*

*6 eggs*

*2 green onions*

*6 oz smoked turkey breast, chopped*

*½ cup blue cheese, crumbled*

*2 Tbsp Blue cheese dressing*

*¼ cup mayonnaise*

*2 Tbsp hot mustard*

*½ rib celery*

Directions:

1. Hard boil the eggs, covered for 12 minutes.

2. In a meanwhile, chop up the smoked turkey breast and the celery.

3. Slice eggs in half lengthwise, scrape the yolks out into a bowl. Add the rest of the ingredients.

4. Grate the green onions over the mixture. Mix all ingredients together.

5. With the tsp fill every egg with the mixture.

6. Place on a serving plate and refrigerate for one hour.

7. Ready! Serve and enjoy!

*[Calories 167 | Total Fats 11.5g | Net Carbs: 0.6g | Protein 14g | Fiber: 0.3 g]*

## Double Cheese Artichoke Dip

[Total Time: 60 MIN| Serve: 12]

*Ingredients:*

*2 cups artichoke hearts, chopped*

*16 oz shredded Mozzarella cheese*

*1 cup grated Parmesan cheese*

*1 cup heavy (whipping) cream*

*1 cup green onion, grated*

Directions:

1. Mix all ingredients together and put in a Slow Cooker.

2. Cook on HIGH mode for about one hour.

3. Sprinkle with chopped green onion, if desired.

*[Calories 227.64 | Total Fats 15g | Net Carbs: 2.32g | Protein 13.67g | Fiber: 1.74g]*

## Easy Artichokes

[Total Time: 2 HR 10 MIN| Serve: 4]

*Ingredients:*

*4 artichokes*

*3 Tbsp lemon juice*

*2 Tbsp coconut butter, melted*

*1 tsp salt and ground black pepper to taste*

*Water*

Directions:

1. Wash and trim artichokes.
2. Start by pulling off the outermost leaves until you get down to the lighter yellow leaves.
3. Then, using a serrated knife, cut off the top third or so of the artichoke.
4. With the same serrated knife, trim the very bottom of the stem.
5. Mix together salt, melted coconut butter, and lemon juice and pour over artichokes.
6. Pour in water to cover artichokes. Cover and cook on LOW 8-10 hours or on HIGH 2-4 hours.
7. Serve and enjoy.

*[Calories 113.58 | Total Fats 6.98g | Net Carbs: 1.56g | Protein 4.29g | Fiber 6.95g]*

## Pancetta 'n' Eggs

[Total Time: 25 MIN| Serve: 4]

*Ingredients:*

*4 large slices Pancetta*

*2 eggs, free-range*

*1 cup ghee, softened*

*2 Tbsp mayonnaise*

*Salt and freshly ground black pepper to taste*

*Coconut oil for frying*

Directions:

1. In a greased non-stick frying pan, bake Pancetta from both sides 1-2 minutes. Remove from the fire and set aside.

2. In a meanwhile boil the eggs. To get the eggs hard-boiled, you need around 10 minutes. When done, wash the eggs with cold water well and peel off the shells.

3. In a deep bowl place ghee and add the quartered eggs. Mash with a fork well. Season it with salt and pepper to taste; add mayonnaise and mix. If you want you can pour in the Pancetta grease. Combine

and mix well. Place the bowl in the fridge for one hour at least.

4. Remove the egg mixture from the fridge and make 4 equal balls.

5. Crumble the Pancetta into small pieces. Roll each ball in the Pancetta crumbles and place on a big platter.

6. Remove the Egg and Pancetta bombs in a fridge for 30 minutes more. Serve cold.

*[Calories 238 | Total Fats 22g | Net Carbs: 0.5g | Protein 7.5g]*

## Parmesan, Herb & Sun-dried Tomato Bombs
[Total Time: 1 HR 20 MIN| Serve: 4]

*Ingredients:*

*1 cup cream cheese*

*1 cup ghee*

*5 Tbsp parmesan cheese*

*¼ cup sun-dried tomatoes, chopped*

*¼ cup Kalamata olives, pitted*

*3 cloves garlic, crushed*

*3 Tbsp herbs mix (basil, parsley, thyme, oregano, parsnip, mint)*

*Salt and freshly ground black pepper to taste*

Directions:

1. In a bowl, combine the cream cheese and ghee. Set aside for 30-45 minutes to soften.

2.  After, mix the ghee and the cream cheese until well combined. Add the chopped Kalamata olives and sun-dried tomatoes.

3.  Add in herbs and crushed garlic; season with salt and pepper to taste. Mix well with the fork and place bowl in the fridge for at least 1 hour.

4.  Remove the cheese mixture from the fridge and create 4 balls. Roll each ball in the grated parmesan cheese and place on a plate.

5.  Return it to the fridge for 30 minutes. Serve and enjoy.

    *[Calories 157 | Total Fats 14g | Net Carbs: 1g | Protein 4.6g | Fiber: 0.5g]*

## Cauliflower Tater Tots

[Total Time: 20 MIN| Serve: 4]

*Ingredients:*

*1 cauliflower head, cut into florets*

*2 oz. mozzarella cheese, shredded*

*¼ cup parmesan cheese, shredded*

*1 organic egg*

*½ tsp garlic powder*

*½ tsp onion powder*

*2 tsp psyllium husk powder*

*Salt and pepper to taste*

*1 cup ghee or lard for frying*

Directions:

1. Steam the cauliflower florets.
2. When done, place them in a food processor and process until you achieve a mash. Set aside.
3. Add the mozzarella, parmesan, egg, and the spices into the mixture. Also, add the psyllium husk and then pulse to combine.
4. Using your hands, roll the mixture into small tater tots sizes.
5. Heat the ghee and then fry until golden brown.
6. Allow cooling for a bit before serving with salsa or sour cream as a dip.

*[Calories 249 | Total Fats 21g | Net Carbs: 4g | Protein 10.3 g | Fiber: 4.5 g]*

## *Keto Margherita Pizza*
[Total Time: 20 MIN| Serve: 2]

*Ingredients:*

*For the crust:*

*2 organic eggs*

*2 tbsp parmesan cheese, grated*

*1 tbsp psyllium husk powder*

*1 tsp Italian seasoning*

*½ tsp salt*

*2 tsp ghee*

*For the toppings:*

*5 basil leaves, roughly chopped*

*2 oz. mozzarella cheese, sliced*

*3 tbsp all-natural tomato sauce*

Directions:

1. Place all the ingredients for the crust in a food processor and pulse until well combined.
2. Pour the mixture into a hot non-stick pan and tilt to spread the batter.
3. Cook until the edges are brown. Flip to the other side and cook for another 45 seconds. Remove from the heat.
4. Spread the tomato sauce on top of the crust, add the mozzarella and basil leaves on top and place in the broiler to melt the cheese for 2 minutes.
5. Serve.

*[Calories 459 | Total Fats 35g | Net Carbs: 3.5g | Protein 27g]*

## *Easy, Peasy, Cheese Pizza*

[Total Time: 35 MIN| Serve: 3]

*Ingredients:*

*2 whole eggs*

*1 cup cheddar cheese, grated*

*1 tbsp psyllium husk*

*3 tbsp pesto sauce*

Directions:

1. Preheat oven to 350$^0$F.

2. Mix eggs and cheese along with the psyllium husk in a bowl and combine well.

3. Place the mixture on baking paper and spread quite thinly. Place in the oven to cook for 15-20 minutes. Remember to keep an eye on it, as it gets brown and crispy quickly relative to the thickness, don't make it too thin.

4. Once cooked, remove from the oven and place whatever you wish over the base, like the pesto sauce or tomato sauce.

5. Top with your favorite pizza toppings such as bacon slices, pepperoni chicken, fresh tomato, and fresh basil.

*[Calories 335 | Total Fats 27g | Net Carbs: 3.2g | Protein 18g]*

## Keto Trio Queso Quesadilla

[Total Time: 20 MIN| Serve: 1]

*Ingredients:*

*¼ cup pepper jack cheese, shredded*

*¼ cup sharp cheddar cheese, shredded*

*1 cup mozzarella cheese, cheese*

*2 tbsp coconut flour*

*1 organic egg*

*½ tsp garlic powder*

*1 tbsp almond milk, unsweetened*

Directions:

1. Set the oven at 350⁰F.

2. Microwave the mozzarella in the microwave until it starts to melt.

3. Allow the mozzarella to cool before adding the coconut flour, egg, garlic powder, and milk.

4. Stir well until you achieve a dough-like consistency.

5. Place the dough in between two parchment papers and roll flat.

6. Remove the top parchment paper, transfer the dough to a baking sheet, and place in the oven to bake for 10 minutes.

7.  Take out from the oven and allow to cool for a few minutes before topping with the cheeses on one-half of the prepared tortilla.

8.  Fold in half and place back in the oven to cook for 5 minutes or until the cheese has melted.

    *[Calories 977 | Total Fats 73g | Net Carbs: 12g | Protein 63g]*

# Bacon and Cheese Melt

[Total Time: 15 MIN| Serve: 2]

*Ingredients:*

*8 pcs string mozzarella cheese sticks*

*8 strips of bacon*

*Olive oil for frying*

Directions:

1.  Preheat your deep fryer to 350$^0$F.

2.  Wrap a cheese stick with one strip of bacon and secure with a toothpick. Repeat until you've used all the bacon and cheese.

3.  Deep fry the cheese sticks in the fryer for 3 minutes. Remove and place on top of a paper towel.

4.  Serve with a leafy green salad on the side.

    *[Calories 590 | Total Fats 50g | Net Carbs: 0g | Protein 34g]*

# Ranch BLT Roll

[Total Time: 10 MIN| Serve: 1]

*Ingredients:*

*4 leaves, romaine lettuce*

*4 bacon strips, cooked and crumbled*

*4 slices deli turkey*

*1 cup cherry tomatoes cut in half*

*2 tbsp mayonnaise*

Directions:

1.   Lay the turkey slice on top of the lettuce leaves.

2.   Spread mayonnaise on the turkey slice and then top with the cherry tomatoes and bacon on top.

3.   Roll the lettuce and then secure with a toothpick.

4.   Serve immediately.

*[Calories 382 | Total Fats 38.5g | Net Carbs: 11.5g | Protein 4.1g | Fiber 6.3g]*

# Portobello Pizza

[Total Time: 25 MIN| Serve: 4]

*Ingredients:*

*1 medium tomato, sliced*

*¼ cup basil, chopped*

*20 pepperoni slices*

*4 Portobello mushroom caps*

*4 oz mozzarella cheese*

*6 tbsp olive oil*

*Black pepper*

*Salt*

Directions:

1. Remove insides of mushrooms and take out meat so that the shell is left.

2. Coat mushrooms with half of oil and season with pepper and salt; broil for 5 minutes then turn over and coat with leftover oil. Bake for an additional 5 minutes.

3. Add tomato to the inside of shell and top with basil, pepperoni, and cheese. Broil for 4 minutes until cheese melts.

4. Serve warm.

   *[Calories 321 | Total Fats 31g | Net Carbs: 2.8g | Protein 8.5g | Fiber 1.3g]*

## Basil and Bell Pepper Pizza

[Total Time: 30 MIN| Serve: 2]

*Ingredients:*

*For Base:*

*½ cup almond flour*

*2 tsp cream cheese*

*1 egg*

*½ tsp salt*

6 oz mozzarella cheese

2 tbsp psyllium husk

2 tbsp parmesan cheese

1 tsp Italian seasoning

½ tsp black pepper

For Toppings:

1 medium tomato, sliced

2/3 bell pepper, sliced

4 oz cheddar cheese, shredded

¼ cup tomato sauce

3 tbsp basil, chopped

Directions:

1. Preheat oven to 400⁰F. Place mozzarella into a microwave safe dish and melt for 1 minute, stirring occasionally.

2. Add cream cheese to melted mozzarella and combine.

3. Mix dry ingredients for base together in a bowl, add egg and combine. Add cheese mixture and use hands to combine into a dough.

4. Form dough into a circle, bake for 10 minutes and remove from oven. Top with tomato sauce, tomato, basil, bell pepper and cheddar cheese.

5. Return to oven and bake for 10 additional minutes.

6. Serve warm.

*[Calories 410 | Total Fats 31.3g | Net Carbs: 5.3g | Protein 24.8g | Fiber 5.8g]*

# Keto Smoothies

## Blueberry Almond Smoothie

[Total Time: 12 MIN| Serve: 2]

*Ingredients:*

*16 oz almond milk, unsweetened*

*1 tsp xylitol*

*4 oz heavy cream*

*¼ cup frozen unsweetened blueberries*

*1 scoop whey vanilla protein powder*

Directions:

1. Put all ingredients in a blender and blend until smooth.

2. Add a little water if it becomes too thick.

3. Measure those blueberries as they add more carbs.

   *[Calories 314 | Total Fats 23.7g | Net Carbs: 8.7g | Protein 16.4g | Fiber: 0.5 g]*

## Choco-Cashew Orange Smoothie

[Total Time: 10 MIN| Serve: 1]

*Ingredients:*

*1 cup cashew milk*

*1 handful of arugula leaves*

*1 tbsp chocolate whey protein powder*

*1/8 tsp orange extract*

*Ice cubes*

Directions:

1.  Place all ingredients in your blender and blend until well united and smooth.

2.  Add extra ice and serve.

    *[Calories 45 | Total Fats 1.05g | Net Carbs: 7g | Protein 3g]*

## *Strawberry Majoram Smoothie*
[Total Time: 10 MIN| Serve: 1]

*Ingredients:*

*¼ cup fresh or frozen strawberries*

*2 fresh marjoram leaves*

*2 tbsp heavy cream*

*1 cup unsweetened coconut milk*

*1 tbsp sugar-free vanilla syrup*

*½ tsp pure vanilla extract*

*Ice cubes*

Directions:

1.  Place all ingredients in your blender and mix until become smooth.

2.  If you wish you can add the ice cubes.

3.  Serve.

    *[Calories 292 | Total Fats 26.7g | Net Carbs: 6g | Protein 2.8g | Fiber: 0.76g]*

## *Low Carb Green Smoothie*

[Total Time: 10 MIN| Serve: 1]

*Ingredients:*

*1 cup almond milk, unsweetened*

*1 cup baby spinach*

*½ ripe avocados*

*½ tbsp stevia*

*1 cup ice*

Directions:

1. Place all the ingredients into a blender and blend until smooth.

2. Serve and consume immediately.

   *[Calories 382 | Total Fats 38.5g | Net Carbs: 11.5g | Protein 4.1g | Fiber 6.3g]*

## *Beet Cucumber Smoothie*

[Total Time: 10 MIN| Serve: 4]

*Ingredients:*

*1 cup spinach leaves*

*2 cups cucumber (peeled, seeded and chopped)*

*½ cup carrot chopped*

*½ cup fresh beetroot*

*¾ cup heavy (whipping) cream*

*4 tsp sweetener of your choice (optional)*

*Handful of ground almonds*

*1 cup ice cubes*

*1 cup water*

Directions:

1.    Place all ingredients in a blender.

2.    Pulse until smooth.

3.    Serve immediately.

*[Calories 137.91 | Total Fats 12.99g | Net Carbs: 3.4g | Protein 1.66g | Fiber: 1.44g]*

### Cilantro and Ginger Smoothie

[Total Time: 10 MIN| Serve: 3]

*Ingredients:*

*½ cup fresh cilantro (chopped)*

*2-inch ginger, fresh*

*1 cucumber*

*2 Tbsp chia seeds*

*½ cup spinach, fresh*

*1 Tbsp almond butter*

*Handful of ground almond*

*1 lime  (or lemon)*

*2 cups water*

Directions:

1.    Blend spinach, cucumber, and water until smooth.

2.    Add the remaining fruits and blend again.

*[Calories 102.72 | Total Fats 6.92g | Net Carbs: 13.96g | Protein 71g | Fiber 6.88g]*


# Green Coconut Smoothie
[Total Time: 10 MIN| Serve: 2]

*Ingredients:*

*1 cup coconut milk*

*1 green apple, cored and chopped*

*1 cup spinach*

*1 cucumber*

*2 Tbsp shaved coconut*

*½ cup water*

*Ice cubes (if needed)*

Directions:

1.  Put all ingredients and ice in a blender; pulse until smooth.
2.  Serve immediately.

*[Calories 216.57 | Total Fats 16.56g | Net Carbs: 8.79g | Protein 2.88g | Fiber: 4g]*

# Green Devil Smoothie
[Total Time: 10 MIN| Serve: 2]

*Ingredients:*

*3 cup kale, fresh*

*½ cup coconut yogurt*

*½ cup broccoli, florets*

*2 celery stalk, chopped*

*2 cup water*

*1 Tbsp lemon juice*

*Ice cubes (if needed)*

## Directions:

1. Blend all ingredients together until smooth and slightly frothy.

   *[Calories 117.09 | Total Fats 4.98g | Net Carbs: 1.89g | Protein 4.09g | Fiber 6.18g]*

## *Green Dream Keto Smoothie*

[Total Time: 10 MIN| Serve: 4]

*Ingredients:*

*1 cup raw cucumber, peeled and sliced*

*4 cups water*

*1 cup romaine lettuce*

*1 cup Haas avocado*

*2 Tbsp fresh basil*

*Sweetener of your choice (optional)*

*Handful of walnuts*

*2 Tbsp fresh parsley*

*1 Tbsp fresh ginger grated*

*Ice cubes (optional)*

Directions:

1.  In a blender, combine all of the ingredients and pulse until smooth.
2.  Add ice if used. Serve cold.

    *[Calories 50.62| Total Fats 3.89g | Net Carbs: 1.07g | Protein 1.1g | Fiber 2.44g]*

## Keto Celery and Nut Smoothie

[Total Time: 10 MIN| Serve: 2]

*Ingredients:*

*2 celery stem*

*1 cup spinach leaves, roughly chopped*

*½ cup pistachio nuts (unsalted)*

*½ avocado, chopped*

*½ cup lime, juice*

*1 Tbsp Hemp seeds*

*1 Tbsp almonds, soaked*

*1 cup coconut water*

*Ice cubes (optional)*

Directions:

1.  Add all ingredients in a blender with a few ice cubes and blend until smooth.

    *[Calories 349.55 | Total Fats 17.88g | Net Carbs: 5.01g | Protein 11.08g | Fiber 9.8g]*

## Lime Peppermint Smoothie
(Total Time: 5 MIN| Serve: 4)

*Ingredients:*

*¼ cup fresh mint leaves*

*¼ cup lime juice*

*½ cup cucumber, chopped*

*1 Tbsp fresh basil leaves, chopped*

*1 tsp chia seed (optional)*

*Handful of chia seeds*

*3 tsp zest of limes*

*Sweetener of your choice to taste*

*1 cup water, divided*

*Ice as needed*

## Directions:

1. Place all ingredients in a blender or food processor.
2. Pulse until smooth well.
3. Fill glasses with ice, pour the limeade into each glass, and enjoy.

   *[Calories 28.11 | Total Fats 1.16g | Net Carbs: 0.75g | Protein 0.84g | Fiber 1.98g]*

## Red Grapefruit Kale Smoothies
[Total Time: 10 MIN| Serve: 4]

*Ingredients:*

*2 cups cantaloupe*

¼ cup fresh strawberries

8 oz coconut yogurt

2 cups kale leaves, chopped

2 Tbsp sweetener of your taste

1 Ice as needed

1 cup water

Directions:

1.   Clean the grapefruit and remove the seeds.

2.   Combine all ingredients in an electric blender and whirl until smooth. Add ice if used and serve.

*[Calories 260.74 | Total Fats 11.57g | Net Carbs: 2.96g | Protein 4.42g | Fiber 7.23g]*

## Simple Keto Avocado Smoothie
[Total Time: 10 MIN| Serve: 2]

*Ingredients:*

*2.6 oz avocado*

*2 cup water*

*2 tsp chia seeds*

*0.5 oz fresh spinach*

*2 fl oz heavy whipping cream*

*1 tsp vanilla extract, unsweetened*

*1 Tbsp extra virgin coconut oil*

*Liquid Stevia extract*

*Few ice cubes*

Directions:

1.  First, bisect the avocado. Carefully remove the seed.

2.  In a blender, put all ingredients, sweetener and the ice (if used) and beat until smooth. Serve.

    *[Calories 226.44 | Total Fats 23.63g | Net Carbs: 0.18g | Protein 1.66g | Fiber 2.86g]*

## Vanilla Protein Smoothie

[Total Time: 5 MIN| Serve: 2]

*Ingredients:*

*1 cup baby spinach*

*5 Tbsp of heavy cream*

*3 Tbsp organic nut butter of your choice*

*½ cup vanilla protein powder*

*3 Tbsp sweetener of your choice*

*1 cup of water*

*Ice cubes*

Directions:

1.  Place all ingredients in a blender and pulse until smooth well.

2.  Serve with ice cubes (optional).

    *[Calories 256.18 | Total Fats 21.79g | Net Carbs: 3.88g | Protein 8.41g | Fiber 4.63g]*

# Almond Choc Shake

[Total Time: 5 MIN| Serve: 2]

*Ingredients:*

*16 oz almond milk, unsweetened*

*1 tbsp chia seeds*

*1 tsp xylitol*

*½ tsp cacao powder*

*4 oz heavy cream*

*1 scoop Whey Chocolate Isolate powder*

*½ cup crushed ice*

Directions:

1. Add all ingredients into the blender and blend until smooth.

   *[Calories 292 | Total Fats 25g | Net Carbs: 4g | Protein 15.27g | Fiber 11.75g]*

# Coco and Blueberry Smoothie

[Total Time: 5 MIN| Serve: 2]

*Ingredients:*

*½ cup blueberries*

*½ cup coconut cream*

*1 tbsp coconut oil*

*½ cup almond milk, vanilla flavor*

*3 ice cubes*

Directions:

1.  Place all the ingredients in a blender and mix until you achieve a smooth consistency.

    *[Calories 237 | Total Fats 21.9g | Net Carbs: 12.1g | Protein 1.9g | Fiber 2.5g]*


# Berry Breakfast Shake
[Total Time: 5 MIN| Serve: 1]

*Ingredients:*

*¾ cup mixed berries*

*1 cup almond milk*

*1 tbsp all-natural peanut butter*

*1 tbsp protein powder*

*¼ tsp cinnamon powder*

*¼ tsp ginger, minced*

Directions:

1.  Add all the ingredients in a blender and blend until smooth.

    *[Calories 319 | Total Fats 15g | Net Carbs: 9g | Protein 28g]*


# Keto Avocado Smoothie
[Total Time: 7 MIN| Serve: 3]

*Ingredients:*

*1 Haas avocado*

*3 oz almond milk, unsweetened*

*3 oz heavy whipping cream*

*6 drops Liquid Stevia*

*Ice cubes*

Directions:

1. Cut the avocado in half, remove the seed and remove the flesh from the skin.
2. In a blender mix the almond milk, avocado, heavy whipping cream, sweetener and ice cubes. Blend 1 minute.
3. Serve.

   *[Calories 252.92 | Total Fats 24.43g | Net Carbs: 8.31g | Protein 3.69g | Fiber: 5.51 g]*

## Caramel Coffee Smoothie
[Total Time: 5 MIN| Serve: 4]

*Ingredients:*

*½ cup heavy cream*

*½ cup almond milk, unsweetened*

*3 Tbsp sugar-free chocolate syrup*

*3 Tbsp sugar-free caramel syrup*

*¾ cup cold coffee*

*2 Tbsp cocoa, unsweetened*

*Ice cubes*

Directions:

1. In a blender add all ingredients and blend until all incorporated well.

2. Pour into glasses and serve.

   *[Calories 170.62 | Total Fats 14.95g | Net Carbs: 9.02g | Protein 2.8g | Fiber 1.92g]*

## Creamy Chocolate Milk

[Total Time: 12 MIN| Serve: 2]

*Ingredients:*

*16 oz almond milk, unsweetened*

*1 tsp xylitol*

*4 oz heavy cream*

*1 scoop whey chocolate isolates powder*

*½ cup crushed ice (optional)*

Directions:

1. Put all ingredients in a blender and blend until smooth.

2. This recipe can be doubled, as can most low carb smoothie recipes.

   *[Calories 292 | Total Fats 25g | Net Carbs: 4g | Protein 15g]*

# Kitchen Measurements

## US Dry Volume Measurements

1/16 tea spoon – dash

1/8 tea spoon – a pinch

3 (three) tea spoons – 1(one) table spoon

1/8 cup – 2 (two) table spoons

¼ (one-quarter)  cup – 4 (four) table spoons

1/3 (one-third) cup – 5 (five) table spoons + 1 (one) tea spoon

½   (half) cup – 8 (eight) table spoons

¾ (three-quarter) cup – 12 (twelve) table spoons

1  (one) cup – 16 (sixteen) table spoons

1 (one) pound – 16 (sixteen)  ounces

## US Liquid Measurements

8 (eight)  fluid ounces – 1 (one) cup

1 (one)  pint – 2 (two) cups (16 fluid ounces)

1 (one) quart – 2 (two)  pints (4 cups)

1 (one)  Gallon – 4 quarts (16 cups)

## Metric to US Conversation

1 (one)  milliliter – 1/5 teaspoon

 5ml – 1 (one)  teaspoon

15 ml – 1 (one) tablespoon

30ml – 1 fluid oz

100ml – 3.4fluid oz

240ml – 1 (one)  cup

*1 (one)  liter – 34 fluid oz*

*1 (one)  liter – 4.2 cups*

*1 liter – 2.1 pints*

*1 liter – 1.06 quarts*

*1 liter - .26 gallon*

*1 gram - .035 ounces*

*100gram – 3.5 ounces*

*500 gram – 1.10 pounds*

*1kilogram – 2.205 pounds*

*1  kilogram – 35oz*

## About the Author

Sandra Woods is a professional chef with 18 years' experience. She is a passionate advocate of ketogenic and anti-aging diets. She emphasis the health benefits of low-carb lifestyle to women and men alike. Her area of expertise includes recipe development, holistic health, and medically restricted diets.

She has authored several books including Home-Made Keto smoothies and juices as well as Home Made Italian Pizza. She runs a successful Keto-based pizza spot called pizza place at Sturbridge, Massachusetts, USA.

80937458R00198

Made in the USA
Lexington, KY
10 February 2018